The White Labyrinth

A Guide
to the Health Care
System

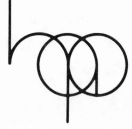

health
administration
press

David Barton Smith
Arnold D. Kaluzny

The White Labyrinth

A Guide to the Health Care System

SECOND EDITION

HEALTH ADMINISTRATION PRESS
Ann Arbor, Michigan
1986

Library of Congress Cataloging-in-Publication Data

Smith, David Barton.
　　The white labyrinth.

　　Bibliography: p.
　　Includes index.
　　1. Medical care—United States. 2. Health services administration—United States. I. Kaluzny, Arnold D. II. Title. [DNLM: Delivery of Health Care—United States. 2. Health Services—Organization & administration—United States. W 84 AA1 S55w]
RA395.A3S65　1986　　　　362.1'0973　　　　86-9859
ISBN 0-910701-13-X

Health Administration Press
1021 East Huron
Ann Arbor, Michigan 48104-9990
(313) 764-1380

To our parents—
Nancy and Henry Smith
and
Helen and Alois Kaluzny—

from whom we learned
not just to see things as they are
and ask why,
but to dream of things that never were
and ask why not.

Contents

Acknowledgments

The actual writing of this second edition was far more chaotic than its final structure may suggest. The first three chapters evolved out of lecture notes and several working papers written by Smith. Chapters 5 and 8 emerged relatively unscathed from the first edition of *The White Labyrinth.* Chapters 4 and 7 were originally drafted by Kaluzny and then reworked by both of us, while chapters 5 and 9 were initially drafted by Smith and then reworked by both of us. The reworking took place through cryptic and sometimes indignant messages between Chapel Hill and Philadelphia. While this distance created difficulties and inefficiencies in completing the project, the insulation it provided us from each other's frustrations no doubt helped to preserve our close friendship, which began 20 years ago in graduate school at The University of Michigan.

Many individuals helped transform these difficulties into an exciting voyage of discovery. On the Philadelphia side, there are more persons than we can possibly mention to whom we owe a debt of gratitude. Particular appreciation is due colleagues Tom Getzen, Irwin Blackstone, and Bob Sigmond, who provided many helpful suggestions on early drafts of chapters. Many former students who are now administrators and health care consultants in the Philadelphia area contributed, often unwittingly, to ideas in the book. Special appreciation in this regard is due Sam Steinberg and Leo Dorazio. Graduate assistants Suzanne Michelle, Luc Zepherin, Elaine Ritter, and Judy Harrington were especially helpful in compiling data and tracking references. We also owe a special debt of gratitude to departmental secretaries Sally Villar and Cindy Gaines, not just for their assistance in preparing initial drafts of the manuscript but for freeing Smith of many day-to-day administrative responsibilities. The study leave granted Smith in 1982 by Temple University provided him time to begin this project and is greatly appreciated. Finally, a special note of appreciation is due Smith's wife, Joan Apt, for her review of the manuscript, for her insights as a practicing administrator, and for her support throughout this project.

On the Chapel Hill side, particular thanks are given to Jean Yates and Donna Cooper, veterans of several previous adventures, who, if not for their intense loyalty and dedication, would have given up in despair. We also want to thank Janice Schopler, Paul A. Kinkel, and Kit Simpson, who joined the writing in its latter phase and added new life and enthusiasm. Kaluzny thanks his chairman, Sagar C. Jain, and other colleagues for their tolerance and support.

Finally, a special joint expression of appreciation is due Daphne Grew and Blair Potter of Health Administration Press for their fine technical assistance and encouragement throughout this project.

Introduction

It has been ten years since we published *The White Labyrinth: Understanding the Organization of Health Care.* In that time there have been dramatic changes in the health care delivery system, changes that are deeply disturbing to persons who struggle with the problems they create. While we were struck by the relevance of *The White Labyrinth*'s original structure to the understanding of those changes, we were made increasingly aware of its limitations. We felt a need to reach further in two directions—toward creating a better conceptual base and toward providing a more concrete explanation of its application.

What began as a revision became an essentially new book. It required (1) a more detailed analysis of the external environmental issues shaping providers, financial as well as regulatory; (2) a more in-depth account of the structural shifts in health care delivery, with both their intended and unintended consequences; and (3) a more detailed presentation of specific operational issues.

As a result, this book is organized into three sections: (1) a description of how the health system was constructed and the consequences of that construction; (2) a description of the organizational mechanisms that underlie its operation; and (3) a detailing of strategies and approaches to change. Each section is divided into three chapters. The first provides a more general description, the second delves into the underlying dynamics, and the third discusses the practical implications. There is also an implicit logical structure to the book: there are three alternative models for structuring organizations (bureaucratic, professional, and participatory) and three levels of analysis (the individual, the organization, and the system as a whole). Were we to be compulsive about this structure, the book would consist of 81 separate subsections (3×3×3×3). It would have all the zip and punch of the *Fed-*

eral Code of Regulations for Medicare, which has possibly done more to accelerate the demise of written communication in the health sector than any other single document. We have chosen a less constrained, more fluid style of presentation, but the reader may find it helpful to be aware of this implicit structure.

The health care system is a labyrinth. Imposing a simplified structure on anything that complex exacts a price. We were unable to include all the rich and diverse empirical and scholarly research that has been carried out over the last ten years. Nor were we able in our examples to develop sufficient detail to provide practitioners with practical procedural guidelines. Instead, we have tried to create a dialogue between research and practice. Such a dialogue requires a temporary suspension of disbelief, which is worthwhile if what is lost in detailed precision is made up for by clarification of underlying issues and relationships. Our aim is to provide a reasonably accurate map of the health care system, the white labyrinth. Any reader who is not conversant with the research literature or administrative practice in health settings will need to supplement this book.

List of Figures and Tables

FIGURES

TABLES

Part I

Creating the Labyrinth

1

Construction

When Alice Cramer became too frail to live by herself, she moved into her son's house. Caring for her at home was costly, and there was no insurance that would cover most of her expenses. She needed to be tube fed, but the food product was costly. Money was tight for her son, an autoworker who had just been laid off. It seemed reasonable to substitute milk. The milk caused diarrhea and dehydration. Reluctantly, the family gave in, and Alice Cramer was admitted, in a weakened condition, to a nursing home.

She did not adjust to her new, unfamiliar surroundings and complained bitterly. Eventually she was admitted to the community hospital, complaining of headaches and abdominal pains. In the hospital she received a complete battery of tests, some unrelated to her symptoms and some whose results were ignored in the treatment regimen that followed. These included three CAT scans, an EEG, and a sinogram, resulting in a laboratory and diagnostic procedure bill that in three weeks totaled over $10,000. Her condition did not improve, and the source of her problems remained unclear. As a last resort, she was referred to a major teaching hospital. A careful workup was conducted, and the doctors concluded that there was nothing basically wrong with her other than the usual frailties of old age, for which medical treatment could do little, and that much of her disorientation and discomfort was related to the testing and drug protocols. After a delay of ten days, the Cramers found a bed in a nursing home across town, and Alice Cramer was sent there. Her health continued to decline, and she died a month later.

Medicare reimbursed those who provided these services to Alice a total of $26,000. The daily cost of the tube feeding that the Cramer family could not afford to pay out of pocket was $6.50.

How could this happen?

Many of the things that happen in health care settings do not make sense from anyone's point of view. The provision of health care has become a labyrinth. Even seasoned professionals sometimes lose their way in it. What once appeared to be a steady march toward health care as a right in this country is now a maze of budget overruns, professionals' self-interest, and regulations. Policymakers are preoccupied with strategies for erecting more effective barriers to the utilization of services rather than tearing them down. The medical profession and the acute-care hospital—assumed after the passage of Medicare and Medicaid to occupy unassailable positions of financial security—are now fraught with uncertainty about which way they should move. They are told they must compete in order to survive. The structure of the health care labyrinth is changing; understanding the changes is not just the key to reducing one's sense of bewilderment, it is the key to both personal and collective survival.

In order to find one's way through the health care labyrinth, one must have a plan. The first step is to understand the health care system. In the first three chapters, we map the development of that system and assess its performance. Once one knows how well the various areas work, one can decide the directions in which one needs to move.

WHY CONSTRUCT A HEALTH SYSTEM?

On a Tuesday morning a Detroit autoworker waits in his HMO's walk-in clinic. The HMO (health maintenance organization) was set up originally by his union to provide comprehensive health care to its members at a fixed cost each year. However, along with many of the others who wait with him, this particular autoworker queues up on Tuesday not for medical care, but to get written justification for his absence from work the day before.

The job of the unskilled autoworker is scarcely designed to instill pleasurable anticipation early Monday morning. Indeed, auto plants have faced serious problems with absenteeism on Mondays and Fridays. The problem is particularly acute during deer season, causing assembly line slowdowns and even threatening to bring entire assembly lines to a halt, something not taken lightly in a city whose economic base has been eroded by the efficiency of Japanese automobile workers.

This creates a frustrating situation for the worker who was legitimately absent on Monday. For one thing, he is likely to receive little sympathy from the medical staff in the clinic and to be dismissed as "another one of the goldbrickers flooding the clinic." As a result, he may come to see the health plan for which his union fought so hard as company medicine. He may even believe that Ford Motor Company and General Motors executives sit on its board. While the idea is patently false, it is not difficult to understand why he might believe this. The physicians are acting as judges, determining whether his deviance (absenteeism) is justified or whether he should have his pay docked.

Every culture has some arrangement for dealing with illness. Though in some cultures the arrangements may be less complex and more intertwined with religion than in ours, they serve a similar function for the society. The health clinic—in fact, the health system as a whole—functions as a mechanism of social control. It shares many similarities with the educational, welfare, and criminal justice systems. Each of these people-processing institutions performs a maintenance function by reducing disruption in the society (Hasenfeld 1983). They do this partly through their efforts at guiding the behavior of individuals into socially desirable directions.

Physicians often act as double agents. They owe allegiance both to the patient and to the larger society in which they practice. A doctor's certification of health or illness may even determine a patient's social or legal fate. When an individual cannot tolerate the demands made on him, as in the example of the autoworker, the physician may end up in the role of arbiter. In such a situation the patient and the physician become either adversaries or conspirators.

All forms of social deviance have certain characteristics in common. First, deviant behavior threatens the effective functioning of the established social order. Second, it is highly skewed; that is, a small percentage of the population accounts for most physician visits, hospital stays, parking violations, tardiness, absenteeism, armed robberies, and so forth. In the Philadelphia Blue Cross plan, for example, subscribers who have at least one alcohol- or drug-related admission to a hospital use eight times as many nondrug- and nonalcohol-related hospital days as other subscribers. As a result, some of the larger employers have developed drug and alcohol programs as a way of controlling the cost of their health insurance benefits (Apt 1984).

Figure 1.1 Flow Chart of Deviance Processing

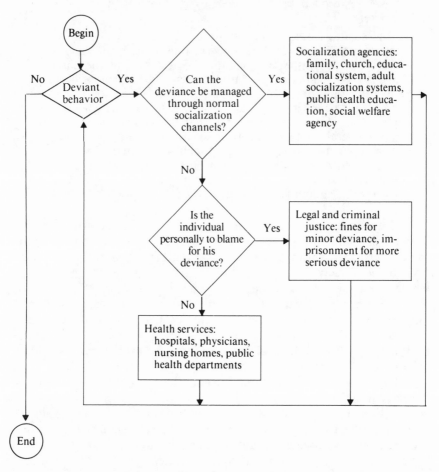

The control of deviance requires specialized deviance-processing institutions—hospitals, prisons, schools. The ways in which deviants are processed through the system are illustrated by the flow chart in figure 1.1. The educational, legal, and health care systems are all part of the larger social maintenance or control system.

Socialization corrects most deviant behavior. Children are trained in appropriate behavior by their families, schools, and other social institutions. When these usual means do not work, how the individual is dealt with depends upon whether or not he is perceived as being individually responsible for his failure. People who collect several hundred parking tickets are generally assumed to be responsible for their own actions. Consequently, they will be prosecuted if and when the law catches up with them. On the other hand, the person who collapses by the side of his car with a heart attack and is rushed to a hospital probably will not be prosecuted for parking illegally.

Deviant individuals may spend a large part of their lives being shuttled among institutions. Where no effective technology exists for eliminating deviance, the processing becomes ritualized.

> A large (over 1,000 beds), prestigious teaching hospital was faced with a problem that occupied much of its legal staff's and chief administrators' time for several weeks. Periodically a man suffering from cerebral palsy, but no other apparent physical illness, showed up in the evening in the emergency room with a variety of physical complaints. Despite admitting the man several times for overnight observation, the medical staff could find no physical basis for his complaints. Consequently, the next time he appeared in the emergency room, the hospital refused to admit him, whereupon he had a temper tantrum in the middle of the large, well-decorated waiting room and proceeded to urinate and defecate on the floor. The physician in charge opted for admission to the short-term psychiatric unit rather than calling the police. The patient was discharged from that unit the next day, after examining physicians concluded that he was not suffering from mental illness but was simply a "manipulative" person.
>
> The individual returned the very next night and reenacted the scene in the waiting room. At this point the administrative staff began pressing for commitment to a state mental hospital. The psychiatrists, however, were uncooperative. They insisted that the man did not have a mental illness that justified institutionalization. He simply had a "dependent, manipulative personality." So the man continued to be passed from the hospital to the police to the psychiatric clinic and back again until everyone involved had lost patience. Finally, the man was committed to a state mental hospital, much to everyone's relief.

Conflict among the various deviance-processing institutions in the health sector over their areas of responsibility, or turf, is inevitable.

HOW CULTURAL VALUES SHAPE THE SYSTEM

Certain values and assumptions, even if not explicitly stated, establish the system's boundaries and shape its development, just as the physical environment imposes constraints on an architect. Health systems, consequently, differ strikingly among countries, even when the technology and resources flowing into those systems are almost identical. Contrast the structure of the Swedish health system with our own.

How Was Sweden's Health Care System Constructed?

The apparent order and elegance of the Swedish health system has long been a source of interest for U.S. visitors. That system contrasts strikingly with the chaos of ownership patterns and the patchwork of reimbursement and regulatory mechanisms in the United States. Efforts have been made, through regional medical programs and health systems agencies, to transplant aspects of that Swedish model to the United States, but with little success.

The Swedish system consists of 23 self-governing counties and municipalities. The governing body of each, the county council, is elected by the public every three years. The medical care board on which council members sit is particularly important, since over 70 percent of the county councils' expenditures are for medical care and related services. These services are financed mainly through a county income tax. The patient pays only a token amount for physician visits and inpatient stays. In counties where there is declining population and a growing proportion of elderly persons, there is revenue sharing from the central government to prevent excessive local tax burdens. The system is structured in an orderly hierarchy that goes from local primary-care centers to district centers, to central facilities, to a regional teaching hospital (Andrews 1973). There is a wide array of services available to individuals who wish to care for a relative in their homes. There are information, referral, and transportation linkages among the elements.

How did this system happen to be created in Sweden? The compulsory national health system was implemented in 1955, but the Swedish health system itself dates to the establishment of regional medical officers in 1668. The real origins may go back even further. Sweden has always been a society in which the protection of the individual against death, disability, and disease was considered a collective, community responsibility. Individuals in local communities were tied together by common and highly risky enterprises (pirating and, later, fishing). In order to ensure the continuation of these enterprises, there had to be a way to make certain that

the families of individuals who failed to return were cared for. In contrast, many settlers of the American colonies were trying to get away from community pressures such as religion, military service, and taxation. Perhaps it should be no surprise that such models of regional delivery have not thrived when transplanted to the United States.

What are the ideological constraints that have shaped the U.S. health care labyrinth? They are invisible. We are only aware of them when we bump into them. They are often not logical and, indeed, are sometimes in conflict with each other. They nonetheless shape the health care labyrinth, even the treatment regimens of individual patients.

A large state psychiatric institution devised a behavior modification unit that had achieved notable success in treating many of the facility's chronic schizophrenic patients. True to the dictums of behavior modification, patients were progressively rewarded for more acceptable behavior. This was done in two ways—through a system of personal privileges and amenities and through an internal economy. A patient who performed at a C or D level received only a bare mattress on the floor of a stark room. Persons on the B level shared comfortably furnished rooms, and A-level people were rewarded with private rooms and payment as a staff aide.

The other set of rewards involved an internal economy based on tokens. Patients were rewarded with tokens for appropriate behavior, such as picking up their rooms, attending group counseling sessions, and participating in group discussions. These tokens could then be used to buy items at the store, including cigarettes and candy. One problem with this system cropped up immediately. A particular patient was constantly stealing tokens from others in the unit. Like many other patients, he was a chain smoker who couldn't accumulate enough tokens to support his habit. Specially marked tokens were made for him to prevent him from continuing his life of crime. Later an even more difficult problem ensued. One patient never used the tokens he accumulated and insisted on giving them away to other patients, subverting his own treatment and that of the unit's other members. As in the first case, specially marked tokens were constructed for him to curb his altruism.

Individuals, institutions, and cultural subsystems must adapt themselves to similar rules for determining how tokens are awarded. One could argue that the rules in the health care sector have swung from awarding tokens for altruism to awarding them for theft. First we will summarize the different ways of defining health care and the conflicting rules of the game implied by each definition; then we will describe how these conflicting definitions have shaped the twists and turns of the health care labyrinth. For the sake of simplicity, we argue that health care can be defined as (1) an economic good, (2) a social relationship, or (3) a professional service.

Health Care As an Economic Good

According to this viewpoint, health care is no different from any other economic good and therefore should operate under the same rules— that is, the rules of the classical model of pure competition. It assumes that health care should be a market where entry is easy, information is accessible to consumers, and prices for services are set by the unrestricted interaction of supply and demand. This is a particularly persuasive model for a society that developed largely in reaction to the imposition of external constraints on the behavior of individuals. There has been, consequently, a long history in this country of antagonism toward any kind of protected status for such services or their practitioners. Echoing popular resistance to state licensure in the nineteenth century, as well as the classical free market position, Friedman argued for the abolition of all forms of professional licensure.

> The American Medical Association is perhaps the strongest trade union in the United States . . . the essence of the power of a trade union is its power to restrict the number who may engage in a particular occupation. . . . Control over admission to medical school and later licensure enables the profession to limit entry. . . .
>
> It is clear that licensure has been at the core of the restriction of entry and that this involves a heavy social cost, both to the individuals who want to practice medicine but are prevented from doing so and to the public deprived of the medical care it wants to buy and is prevented from buying. Let me now ask the question: Does licensure have the good effects that it is said to have?
>
> In the first place, does it really raise standards of competence? . . . The rise of the professions of osteopathy and of chiropractic is not unrelated to restriction of entry into medi-

cine. On the contrary, each of these represented, to some extent, an attempt to find a way around restriction of entry. Each of them, in turn, is proceeding to get itself licensed and to impose restrictions. . . . These alternatives may well be of lower quality than medical practice would have been without the restrictions on entry into medicine. . . .

Trained physicians devote a considerable part of their time to things that might be done by others. The result is to reduce drastically the amount of medical care. The relevant average quality of medical care, if one can at all conceive of the concept, cannot be obtained by simply averaging the quality of care that is given; that would be like judging the effectiveness of a medical treatment by considering only the survivors; one must allow for the fact that restrictions reduce the amount of care. The result may well be that the average level of competence in a meaningful sense has been reduced by the restrictions. . . .

Suppose that anyone had been free to practice medicine without restriction except for legal and financial responsibility for any harm done to others through fraud and negligence. I conjecture that the whole development of medicine would have been different. The present market for medical care, hampered as it has been, gives some hints of what the difference would have been. Group practice in conjunction with hospitals would have grown enormously. Instead of individual practice plus large institutional hospitals conducted by government or eleemosynary institutions, there might have developed medical partnerships or corporation-medical teams. . . . These medical teams—department stores of medicine, if you will—would be intermediaries between the patients and the physician. Being long-lived and immobile, they would have a great interest in establishing a reputation for reliability and quality. For the same reason, consumers would get to know their reputation. They would have specialized skill to judge the quality of physicians; indeed, they would be the agent of the consumer in doing so, as the department store is now for many a product . . . the great argument for the market is its tolerance of diversity, its ability to utilize a wide range of special knowledge and capacity. It renders special groups impotent to prevent experimentation and permits the customer, not the producers, to decide what will serve the customers best (Friedman 1962, 150–60).

What is particularly striking, as will be seen in the next chapter, is how much closer we have come to developing a system along those lines.

While most physicians are horrified by such arguments, both physicians and other providers have used similar arguments to combat government interference in their professions and institutions. Those who choose to live by the sword of the marketplace may die by it as well.

There are even more worrisome aspects of this approach to health care. It applies to human beings the same criteria it uses to govern the maintenance and replacement of machines. Once the costs of maintenance exceed the costs of replacement, the machine or individual is scrapped. Traditionally, the costs and benefits of providing health services have been calculated by the "human capital" method. Although there are a variety of refinements on this method, it basically involves calculating the present net value of the future earnings of a given individual or group (by age, sex, or economic status) in order to arrive at the dollar value of a life. The identical method is used in making capital investment decisions in industry.

As indicated in figure 1.2, human lives do not have equal economic value. If we calculate the present value of future income for people at different ages, we find that men are worth more than women and that children and the elderly are worth far less than middle-aged individuals. Recently a method that is more compatible with the values of the classical competitive market has been developed; this method is referred to as the "willingness-to-pay" method (Landefeld and Seskin 1982). In it, the individual is asked to set the price he or she would be willing to pay in order to reduce his or her risk of death or disability. This approach gets away from valuing life simply on the basis of future income lost, but, since these decisions will be based largely on individual income, it is doubtful that the overall picture would differ much from that shown in figure 1.2.

It is interesting to note that, in the human capital method (and perhaps implicit in the willingness-to-pay method), as the discount rate or interest rate associated with such investments goes up, the value of human life drops. Health is a long-term investment, particularly for the young. The value of long-term investments drops as the interest rate or discount rate rises. Perhaps the growing resistance to investment in both public and private health insurance programs is directly related to the rise in interest rates.

Not only is the willingness to invest down, but investment is becoming more selective.

In a lush area just outside the metropolitan sprawl, stands the white marble corporate headquarters building of a major oil company. Off its air-conditioned courtyard filled with

Figure 1.2   Present Value of Lifetime Earnings, by Sex and Discount Rate, 1980

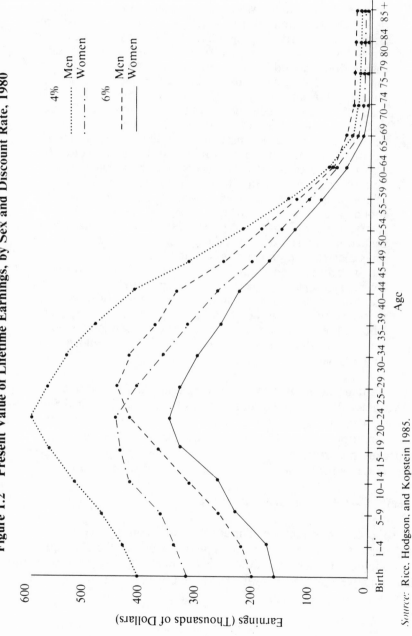

Source: Rice. Hodgson. and Kopstein 1985.

greenery is a suite devoted to the executive exercise program. Top executives who are identified as essential to the corporation (especially those whose free annual physical examinations suggest their health is at risk) are selected for the program. An exercise program designed by an exercise physiologist in conjunction with a physician is developed for each individual and is closely monitored and altered depending on blood pressure, pulse readings, and measures of body fat. Diet assistance is provided. The executives' exercise routines, blocked into their schedules by their secretaries, consist of a series of exercise stations designed to alternately develop aerobic capacity and muscular strength. The exercises are performed before a full-length mirror in front of a color television, where each individual can watch the videotaped public television show of his choice. Treadmills are used instead of a jogging track, since it was discovered that the executives found it hard to maintain their assigned pace—each tended to try to get ahead of the others. Now they can jog beside each other at speeds individually regulated by the exercise physiologist. The program is justified because of the substantial investment the company has made in these top executives and because the cost of replacing them would come to many times their annual salaries. One of the jobs of some of these executives is to delay and modify the air pollution controls imposed on their refineries, controls based largely on estimates of what different levels of pollution would cost in human lives.

Similar reasoning may support what appears to be the increasingly less aggressive enforcement of standards by the Occupational Safety and Health Administration (Greenberg 1982). Perhaps as a result of this preoccupation with the economic value of human life, our society tends to isolate and segregate economically "useless" people into retirement, ghettoes, nursing homes, and the back wards of state institutions.

Health Care As a Social Relationship

In spite of the attraction of individualistic, competitive market rules, American society has never been able to accept all the consequences of imposing such rules on health care. Although we may attempt to insulate ourselves, as Slater (1970) has noted, we are not indifferent to the effects.

Our ideas about institutionalizing the aged, psychotic, retarded, and infirm are based on a pattern of thought that we might call the "Toilet Assumption"—the notion that unwanted matter, unwanted difficulties, unwanted complexities and obstacles will disappear if they are removed from our immediate field of vision—we throw the aged and psychotic into institutional holes where they cannot be seen. Our approach to social problems is to decrease their visibility: out of sight, out of mind . . . when these discarded problems rise to the surface again—a riot, a protest, an exposé in the mass media—we react as if a sewer had backed up. We are shocked, disgusted, and angered and immediately call for the emergency plumber (the special commission, the crash program) to insure that the problem is once again removed from consciousness (Slater 1970, 15).

In reaction to the darker, more alienating implications of the market view of health care, we swing toward the other extreme, toward defining health care as something completely outside the normal economic sphere. Its function is "social maintenance" rather than "capital maintenance": the creation of a sense of social solidarity, of a cooperative human community. It requires an open-ended social commitment to meet all the health care needs of all the individuals in that society. It is not surprising, then, that national health services and insurance initiatives that would assure more equitable access to health care have appeared in the United States and other developed countries during or shortly after major wars, which require collective sacrifices. The notion of adequate health care as a right in the Medicare and Medicaid legislation came at the same time that the Vietnam War was escalated. It is given at least lip service in the mission statements of most health services institutions and professional associations in the United States.

Health Care As a Professional Service

The Great American Dream: to serve humanity
and make a 40 percent profit on the side.

A society that views health care as both an economic good and a social relationship is, like the patient in the back ward, schizoid. How does one incorporate both of these perspectives into a stable, workable synthesis? One need not actually resolve the underlying conflict; one can simply create some myths that will do it. The task of reconciling these contradictions is, consequently, delegated to the health care "professions" (primarily medicine) and to "science." The health care professions subsume both the notion of health care as an economic good and the notion of health care as a special social relationship. Society gives the professions special status: they can restrict and control entry, and they can police themselves. In exchange, society delegates certain responsibilities to the professions. The health care professions are to foster that social relationship, through adherence to professional ethics and values, while at the same time they are to provide an economic good.

Society's faith in the ability of the health care professions to reconcile these conflicts is strengthened by the scientific and technological basis of those professions. Perhaps the best way to resolve, or at least to believe one has resolved, basic conflicts between different sets of values is to redefine the conflicts as technical rather than social problems. Thus, one can focus on basic and applied research for the elimination of disease and disability even though effective preventive treatment is already well understood. Similarly, one can focus on the problems of eliminating abuse in a Medicaid program through the development of computerized medical information systems. Neither approach does much to resolve the underlying conflicts in how resources are utilized and for whose benefit; however, transforming social problems into technical problems that are amenable to solution helps to mitigate social tensions and, at least to some degree, serves both the capital and social maintenance functions of the health care system.

CONSTRUCTION OF THE HEALTH CARE SYSTEM

The health care system is designed to incorporate these contradictory definitions of health care, or rules of the game. It has changed from an organizationally simple system into a labyrinth in the last 60 years. (The major elements of the system are shown in figure 1.3.) In the remainder of this chapter, we discuss the transformations that have taken place among primary providers—that is, those individuals and organizations directly involved in the provision of health services (for example, public health agencies, physicians, hospitals and related institutions, and the allied health professions). The relationships among these primary providers, the financing mechanisms, secondary providers, and consumers will be discussed in greater detail in the next chapter, which focuses on the current operation of the system. We will touch briefly in this chapter on some of the historical developments in the financial arrangements supporting primary providers, because these developments are intimately related to the changes in organization of primary providers.

Figure 1.3 Major Elements of the Health Care System

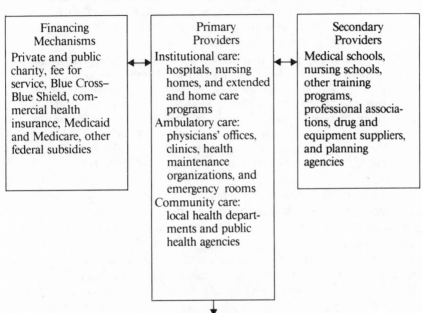

Source: Kelman 1973.

Creation of the Public Health Sector

Here are a few citations [from the *Report of the Council of Hygiene and Public Health of the Citizens Association of New York upon the Sanitary Condition of the City*] which indicate the state of our own metropolitan city of New York as late as 1865.

Of the Sixth Ward an inspector says, "Domestic garbage and filth of every kind is thrown into the streets, covering their surface, filling the gutters, obstructing the sewer culverts, and sending forth perennial emanations which must generate pestiferous disease. In winter the filth and garbage, etc., accumulate in the streets to the depth sometimes of two or three feet." In the Thirteenth Ward "the streets are generally in a filthy and unwholesome condition; especially in front of the tenant houses, from which the garbage and slops are, to a great extent, thrown into the streets, where they putrefy, rendering the air offensive to the smell and deleterious to health.

The refuse of the bedrooms of those sick with typhoid and scarlet fevers and smallpox is frequently thrown into the streets, there to contaminate the air, and, no doubt, aid in the spread of those pestilential diseases."

... It was estimated that 18,000 persons were living in cellars in New York at this time; and in the Fourth Ward many of these cellar dwellings were below high-water mark. "At high tide the water often wells up through the floors, submerging them to a considerable depth. In very many cases the vaults of privies are situated on the same or a higher level, and their contents frequently ooze through the walls into the occupied apartments beside them" (Winslow 1923, 9–10).

The public health sector emerged in response to such conditions. The fervor with which it identified health care as a social relationship bordered on the evangelical. In the mid-nineteenth century, the average life expectancy for the gentry in England was 36 years; it was only 16 years for the laboring class. Life expectancy in Boston and most other American cities at this time was somewhat less. The Shattuck report of 1841 documented conditions in Massachusetts and recommended the creation of state and local boards of health, sanitary inspectors, collection and analysis of statistics, and preventive medicine and health promotion (Shattuck, Banks, and Abbott 1850). Local health departments with full-time staff began to develop in the last half of the nineteenth century; their activities have since blended into those of state health departments and federal agencies responsible for public health activities.

The public health movement, in spite of opposition from local medical societies, lack of knowledge of the etiology of many diseases, and limited financial resources, made impressive gains between 1850 and 1920. Life expectancy increased; infant and crude mortality rates dropped as public health measures brought infectious diseases under control; and a general rise in income and standard of living contributed to improved health status. The prediction of nineteenth-century reformers that improvement of social conditions would achieve more rapid results than advances in medical science was clearly demonstrated by World War I.

To state that the death rate of New York City has been reduced from 25 per 1000 in 1890 to 13 per 1000 in 1920 may perhaps leave one unmoved; but think for a moment what such statistics mean in terms of human life and human happiness. Today in that great city there are 201 death beds every twenty-four hours. If the death rate of thirty years ago were still in force there would be 384—a savings of 183 lives with each revolution of the earth. If death be the wage of sanitary sin, nearly one half the debt has been remitted in a period of thirty years. . . .

If we had but the gift of second sight to transmute abstract figures into flesh and blood, so that as we walk along the street we could say "That man would be dead of typhoid fever," "That woman would have succumbed to tuberculosis," "That rosy infant would be in its coffin"—then only should we have a faint conception of the meaning of the silent victories of public health. For such achievements we may thank God and take courage for the future, bearing on our banners that eternal phrase of Cicero: "In no single thing do men approach the Gods more nearly, than in the giving of safety to mankind" (Winslow 1923, 64–65).

The charismatic crusaders are gone now, and public health agencies appear to be moving further and further into the background, stepping back deferentially for local hospitals and physicians wherever feasible. Public health agencies are now the provider of last resort. It is only when "the sewer backs up," in Slater's phrase—when there is a Love Canal, a Legionnaires' disease, an AIDS epidemic, or a nuclear accident —that we get a taste of the political controversy, the excitement of unraveling a mystery, and the widespread public fear that surrounded public health activities earlier in this century. What began as a social and political movement for reform became a procedure-oriented, cumbersome, low-profile bureaucracy.

Evolution of the Medical Profession

Medical practitioners, in contrast to public health practitioners, embraced early on the notion of health care as an economic good. Colonial America, according to one early observer, was "free of the three great scourges of mankind—priests, lawyers and physicians" (Ebert 1973, 183). It was a long, uphill battle for the medical profession to carve out a position of special privilege. In the age of "heroic medicine" (roughly 1780 to 1850), warring cults sprang up in opposition to the standard practices of bleeding and dosing with calomel. There were no restrictions on the practice of medicine: anyone could prescribe medication and a regimen for the ill. In the early nineteenth-century Jacksonian era of revolt against privilege, cults of all kinds flourished without restraint. Many attempted to define health care in terms of broader social relationships. The Thomsonians, for example, followed the teachings of an itinerant herbalist who was influential perhaps because his herbal potions did less damage than the more powerful chemical doses of the traditionalists, and perhaps because he taught self-care and that women should be the primary providers of medical care for their families. The Thomsonians' reaction against orthodox medicine has resurfaced in the current self-help and holistic health movements.

Traditional practitioners spent much of their energy fighting "quackery." Members of the allopathic group in 1847 founded the American Medical Association (AMA) and continued their efforts to control medical education and restrict the practice of medicine to persons who practiced as they did. The only significant present-day survivors of those sectarian battles with the AMA are the osteopaths, who, while originally emphasizing manipulation of the joints, are now almost indistinguishable from allopathic physicians. They have, however, by their willingness to undertake separate negotiations for payment under Medicare and their long-standing focus on family practice, prevented allopathic physicians from monopolizing American medicine (Blackstone 1977).

By 1900 the AMA had succeeded in gaining some restrictions on the practice of medicine, although sellers of nostrums and practitioners of all sorts still flourished. Over 150 medical schools still granted degrees to students who completed curricula of dubious and wildly varied content. In 1904, the Council on Medical Education was created in an effort to direct professional education along more scientific lines. In the same era, leaders of the AMA, many of whom were scientists and educators rather than practitioners, allied themselves with the Carnegie and Rockefeller foundations in the struggle to bring order to the chaotic medical scene. The Carnegie Foundation commissioned a study, the Flexner report, published in 1910, which became a landmark in the development of American medical education and practice.

The Flexner report set the pattern for four-year postgraduate training of doctors in an academic setting. As a result of the report, marginal medical schools closed and medical education became firmly rooted in university graduate education. By 1922, the number of medical schools dropped to 82; the number of graduates and the ratio of physicians to population also fell abruptly. The scientific basis of medical practice was firmly established with impressive financial support from philanthropic foundations, later greatly extended by public funds (Berliner 1975).

Four drastic changes were made in medical practice between 1900 and 1922: (1) entry to the profession was greatly restricted, leading to enhanced prestige and income for the professional practitioner; (2) specialists replaced general practitioners as advances were made in scientific medicine; (3) health manpower, which in pre-Flexner days had consisted almost entirely of physicians, became a physician elite assisted by nurses and allied workers; and (4) the medical profession emerged as a homogeneous and powerful group that was much more insulated from competitive market pressures. These changes brought about changes in health facilities, financing, and all other sectors of the health care system.

Modern medical practice is almost the mirror image of what it was in 1900. A single, homogeneous profession exercises a virtual monopoly over the provision of services, rather than a large and colorful array of practitioners competing against each other. While in 1900 over 90 percent of physicians were general practitioners, today little more than 10 percent are. Twenty percent of physicians now work in group practice or hospital-based settings, and most earn a large proportion of their incomes from the hospital-based portion of their practices. In 1900, group practice was unheard of, and practitioners' services in hospitals were largely given free.

The very success of this transformation has built up pressure to move in the opposite direction. The growing investment of public funds in medical schools produced pressure for expanded enrollments. By 1990, the physician-to-population ratio is projected to be about 250 per 100,000, in contrast to the 160 per 100,000 in 1900. With this increase in the supply of physicians has come a shift away from the overstocked specialty practices toward family and general practices. The house call, the predominant form of service offered by physicians in 1900 and until recently considered extinct, is staging a comeback. Some observers predict that this increased supply of physicians will shift physicians' practice patterns away from hospitals and that hospitals will increasingly find themselves in direct competition with physicians. Nurse practitioners have entered the struggle for recognition as independent practitioners and have won some modest victories in a few states. In many communities, holistic health centers have sprung up, combining the preventive, spiritual, holistic aspects of treatment practiced by some nineteenth-century "cults"—aspects considered lost in twentieth-century medicine.

All of these changes in how physicians practice have been shaped by how physicians are paid. At the turn of the century, physicians (at least those practicing in major metropolitan areas) divided their practice between their private, paying patients, usually cared for in the patients' own homes, and the charitable care they gave in voluntary or municipal hospitals. In this way physicians reconciled the economic good and social relationship definitions of health care. Physicians attempted to balance the free care they gave with payments from private patients, based on their ability to pay. This Robin Hood principle, disdainfully viewed by many economists today as "cross-subsidization," became embedded in the patterns of payment for health services. This principle can be found today in the sliding fee schedules of most Blue Shield plans and in the hidden subsidies that self-paying or self-insured patients provide for public assistance patients in hospitals. Originally, physicians' charitable activities were to some extent repaid by the status accorded them and by the opportunity to be connected with teaching facilities, thereby continuing their own professional development.

While most physicians charged their private patients fees, other methods for payment existed. One such method was capitation, which was particularly common among recent European immigrants. A physician would contract to provide care for members of a fraternal lodge and would be paid a flat rate each year based on the number of members. Given the large number of struggling physicians that existed around 1900, the lodges were in an ideal position to negotiate low prices and reasonable service for their members. (One variant of such practices, discounted fees for lodge members, has recently resurfaced as the preferred provider organization.) Not surprisingly, such practices were viewed with hostility by local medical societies, and their concerted efforts resulted in the elimination of such arrangements before 1920 (Rosen 1977). The hostility of organized medicine toward capitation payment, as illustrated by the Ross-Loos Medical Group's battles with a local medical society, has continued until quite recently, when new packaging and concessions to physician control and profit sharing have muted much of their resistance.

The Saga of the
Ross-Loos Medical Group

In April of 1929, the Ross-Loos Medical Group opened in Los Angeles. The group provided comprehensive medical care on a prepaid basis for 1,500 employees of the county Department of Water and Power and their families. Enrollment swelled to 12,576 by 1935. The growth of the clinic, however, coincided with the onset of the Depression, and opposition within the county medical society grew. Local physicians experienced rapid declines in income. It is doubtful that the Ross-Loos plan actually took many paying patients away from private practitioners, since the income group serviced by the plan would have been unable to foot substantial medical bills without the risk pooling which the plan made possible. Nevertheless, concrete economic difficulties, combined with the ambiguous threat of a form of practice labeled "socialistic and Communistic" by organized medicine, made concerted opposition within the county medical society inevitable. Drs. Ross and Loos were asked to appear to discuss the alleged unethical solicitation of patients. With little attempt at a judicious examination of the facts, they were summarily discharged from the society.

The expulsion became a national cause célèbre. In 1933 there was fear of a rising tide of support for a compulsory federal health insurance program. The state association refused to overrule the county society, and the fight was carried to the AMA judicial council. An unfavorable ruling by the council would lead to a court trial likely to attract enormous unfavorable attention to organized medicine. After lengthy deliberation, the council chose to rule that Ross and Loos had not had a fair trial and therefore should be reinstated rather than pass on the merits of their type of practice. Harassment at the local level, however, did not end. Applications for county medical society membership of new physicians in the Ross-Loos group were not acted upon, making it impossible for them to gain staff privileges at better hospitals. The threat of Justice Department action against the AMA for its activities related to other prepaid group practices brought about a "peaceful" settlement, and the physicians' applications were duly accepted.

By 1939, Dr. Loos was sitting on the council of the county medical society, and Dr. Ross had come to hold several important committee assignments. Organized medicine and the two physicians had learned to live peacefully with each other. In 1939, the California Medical Association launched a prepayment plan for physicians, the nation's first Blue Shield plan, modeled after the experience of Ross and Loos. Loos served as spokesman for organized medicine, opposing the national health insurance drive in the early 1950s (Kisch and Viseltear 1967, 1–37; paraphrased).

The predominant form of payment remains fee-for-service, and it would be a mistake to underestimate its impact on the provision of services. Other forms of payment appear to encourage physicians to become a good deal more conservative and concerned with preventing heroic medical intervention. The consequences of such incentives will be discussed at length in the next chapter. It is sufficient to point out here that physicians have so far successfully controlled how they are paid and what they can charge. Blue Shield programs were developed by medical societies as a defense against the development of other insurance schemes that might erode such control. The passage of the Medicare and Medicaid legislation in 1965 and subsequent administration of those programs have largely protected physicians' control. For example, under part B of Medicare, physicians can be paid what is "usual and customary" in their region. They may submit whatever fees they choose for reimbursement, but Medicare will not reimburse them directly for any amount above a certain percentile in the distribution of fees for similar services submitted previously by all physicians in the region. The fees they submit, however, will be used in computing a payment ceiling for a subsequent year. If this seems onerous, physicians can simply refuse Medicare assignment and bill their patients directly for whatever they like. It is then up to the patient to obtain reimbursement from Medicare for the allowable charges and to make up the difference. Efforts to freeze fees and discourage physicians from refusing assignment, however, began in earnest in 1984.

State welfare Medicaid programs have been less generous and have imposed far more restrictive ceilings on payments. Many physicians have found it easier to refuse to participate in them, however, than to refuse to provide free care. The increased competition brought about by more physicians and more prepaid schemes will probably curtail the individual physician's freedom to control his own working conditions and income. In some ways, we may indeed be coming full circle to the situation in 1900, when physicians were in a far weaker bargaining position.

The Transformation of Hospitals and Related Institutions

— A hospital in Atlanta, with identical twin towers connected by a single corridor, each with separate, identical laboratory, dietary, and operating rooms—facilities completed in the 1950s, when separate could still pass as equal.

— A hospital in the Bronx serving kosher food to its patients, 70 percent of whom are black.

— A large hospital in Manhattan still using the remnants of separate sets of china and silverware for the private, semiprivate, and ward units.

Figure 1.6   Change in Utilization of General Hospitals in the United States During Selected Years, 1928–1978

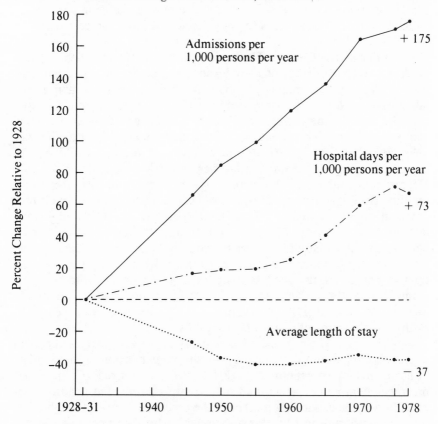

Note: For 1928, this includes all hospitals except tuberculosis and psychiatric hospitals; for 1946–78, it includes all nonfederal short-term general and other special hospitals listed by the American Hospital Association.

Adapted from: Donabedian, Axelrod, and Wyszewianski 1980, 81.

the growth in number of short-term public hospital beds has been substantially less.

Overall, as indicated in figure 1.6, hospital admissions per 1,000 persons have risen 175 percent since 1931, and the number of hospital days per 1,000 persons has risen more than 73 percent. Dramatic drops in average length of stay since the introduction of the Medicare prospective payment system have accentuated the shift toward greater intensity of hospital services. Since 1946, the ratio of full-time staff to patients has increased more than threefold, and the cost per admission has increased fifteenfold. Most of the changes that have taken place since the 1930s, however, were stimulated more by the changing patterns of payment for hospital services than by the accreditation process itself.

Financing the Change. The rapid growth and development of hospitals and related institutions would not have taken place without adequate financing. The majority of patients in many metropolitan hospitals were treated free of charge as late as 1917 (Rosner 1982). Charitable contributions to these local community institutions were their major source of income. The Great Depression threatened to stall further development indefinitely. Private and public philanthropy could not be depended upon to sustain development, and few patients during the Depression could afford the increasing cost of hospital care. Recognizing this, Baylor University Hospital in Dallas, Texas, worked out a prepayment plan with area teachers. The idea caught on quickly, and similar voluntary community hospital insurance programs—Blue Cross plans—sprung up rapidly all over the country. The new insurance plans faced almost no opposition, since hospitals viewed them as a more attractive source of financial security than government insurance programs. Just as the subsequent Blue Shield programs assured a relatively high degree of control for physicians, so the Blue Cross plans seemed to assure a high degree of control for hospitals.

World War II wage and price controls, along with increased collective bargaining in industry, resulted in a rapid expansion in the number of health insurance benefit packages offered to employees. Commercial insurance companies, which had not previously provided health insurance, joined the expanding market in the early 1950s, even though there was a concurrent effort to pass a national health insurance bill. Debate concerning the appropriate role of each of these insurance mechanisms (voluntary, commercial, and public) continues unabated. In essence, it represents a continuation of the conflict between what health care represents and the rules that should apply to the provision of it. The arguments center on four questions, which will be outlined below.

First, to what extent should an insurance program be mandated for patients and providers alike? Physician groups opposed to the passage of national health insurance legislation after World War II made their position clear:

Awake America!
During the last twelve years we have witnessed the encroach-

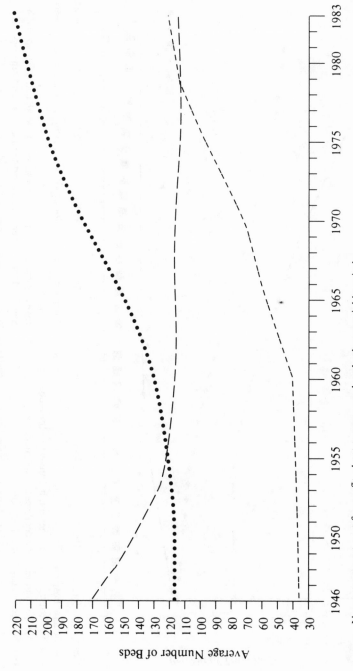

Figure 1.4   Size of Acute-Care Hospitals, by Type of Hospital, 1946–1983

Average Number of Beds

220
210
200
190
180
170
160
150
140
130
120
110
100
90
80
70
60
50
40
30

1946   1950   1955   1960   1965   1970   1975   1980   1983

••• Nongovernment, not-for-profit, short-term general and other special hospitals
—   Investor-owned (for-profit), short-term general and other special hospitals
– – State and local government, short-term general and other special hospitals

Source: American Hospital Association 1984.

Figure 1.5 Breakdown of Total U.S. Hospital Beds, by Type of Hospital, 1948–1983

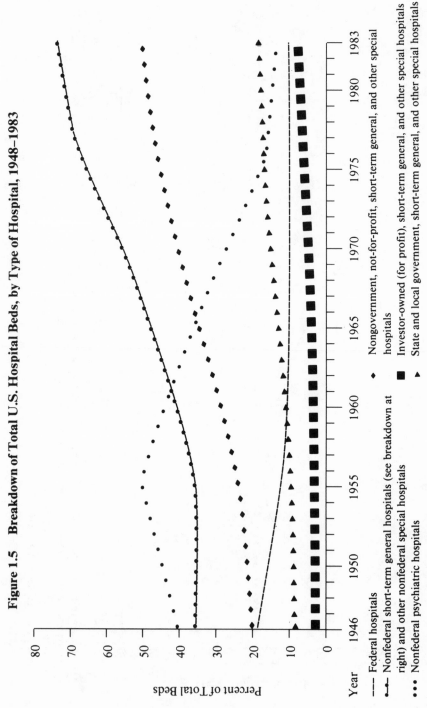

Year

Percent of Total Beds

— Federal hospitals

•—• Nonfederal short-term general hospitals (see breakdown at right) and other nonfederal special hospitals

••• Nonfederal psychiatric hospitals

• Nongovernment, not-for-profit, short-term general, and other special hospitals

◆ Investor-owned (for profit), short-term general, and other special hospitals

■ State and local government, short-term general, and other special hospitals

Source: American Hospital Association 1984.

ments that are leading, even now, to a creeping paralysis of our social and economic functions. . . . The designs of schemers is [sic] made crystal clear. It is not merely a matter of medical care—or the regimentation of the medical profession—that is at stake. It is our Country—our beliefs, our concepts—our very souls that are involved.

The physicians and dentists of this country—to a greater degree and extent than any other groups—have taken time to understand, appraise and vigorously wage an all-out war against this menace. They have alerted millions of people.

The time has now come when every American—every believer in the American Way of Life—should join in unqualified opposition to this attempt to foist on this country this foreign ideology—this strictly Collectivist mechanism—Compulsory Health Insurance (National Physicians Committee 1946, 8).

Resistance to external controls has created convoluted yet pragmatic compromises in all health insurance programs. Whether a completely voluntary system can be made to work is a matter of ongoing debate.

Second, should hospitals be paid on the basis of what it costs them to provide specific services or on the basis of a negotiated charge? Often in actual situations, costs are defined as "allowable costs" and charges are defined as "reasonable costs," and the distinctions between the two forms of reimbursement become blurred. Nevertheless, the approach adopted can have important long-run consequences, as will be described in chapter 2. In the early Blue Cross plans, hospitals were paid the fixed daily rate, or charge, that they were accustomed to receiving from their private patients. In the late 1940s, this approach fell into disfavor, since Blue Cross plans had become increasingly concerned with paying only what it cost to produce a service and hospitals were attracted to a system of payment that would assure allowances for capital and patient care improvements. We appear to be coming full circle, since increasing interest is being expressed in what are essentially charge-based systems—or "prospective reimbursement" systems, as they are now labeled. The most recent trend, diagnosis-related groups (DRGs) for Medicare recipients, extends such systems one step further, paying a fixed charge for each admission in a particular diagnostic category, regardless of the actual number of days the patient is hospitalized. Such payment systems offer vastly different incentives to hospitals. It is possible, though, that we may be trading our current problem of spiraling costs for the older problem of assuring a reasonable standard of care.

Third, how should the actual hospitalization costs of insured individuals and groups be paid? Should they simply be averaged across all subscribers in a community, or should they be related to the likelihood that the particular individual or group will need costly services? The ideal of the original Blue Cross plans was community rating. That is, every individual or employer in a given community would pay the same amount, regardless of risk. This would, in theory, enable everyone to obtain coverage at a reasonable rate. The approach was foreign to the commercial insurance companies that entered the health insurance market after World War II. Commercial insurers began to lure low-risk groups away from Blue Cross plans, offering lower, experience-based ratings. This "skimming the cream," as the practice was called by those who believed that community rating provided a way to meet health insurance needs within a voluntary framework, contributed to the demise of the community rating approach. In order to defend their shares of the market, most Blue Cross plans followed suit; Medicare and Medicaid later filled part of the resulting gap.

The issue resurfaced when HMOs began to set rates. In order to attract subscribers, rates for the more comprehensive health insurance packages offered by HMOs must be set at approximately the same level as traditional hospital insurance packages. The ability of some HMOs to maintain low rates while remaining financially viable has been a focus of ongoing debate. That is, are these HMOs skimming the cream from Blue Cross and commercial enrollments, or are they efficient enough to support the broader benefit packages at rates equivalent to conventional hospital insurance alone?

Finally, what should the respective roles of the voluntary, commercial, and public health insurance mechanisms be? Any major reforms in the financing of health services will favor one or another of these mechanisms. Some of the game playing and jockeying for position will be described in the next chapter. Each of these mechanisms is entrenched in the existing system of health care financing, making any major change that would erode its position far more difficult now than it would have been 60, 40, or even 20 years ago.

The Transformation of Health Manpower

Changes in the health care work force in this century have mirrored changes in the organizations where health care workers are employed. These changes also reflect more general changes produced by industrialization. The year 1910 marked another milestone besides the Carnegie Foundation–supported Flexner report and related improvements in scientific medicine. It marked a basic shift in the organization of work and the structure of jobs, a shift graphically illustrated in Carnegie's own steel industry. We will describe that shift in detail, since the basic changes in the organization of work in the health sector since 1910 seem to have followed a similar pattern.

Between 1890 and 1910, steel replaced iron as the building block of industrial society, and the United States surpassed Great Britain as the major steel producer in the world (Stone 1974, 116). Carnegie consolidated his steel-producing empire in the 1890s, and shortly afterwards formed the world's first billion-dollar corporation, United States Steel. At its inception, U.S. Steel controlled 80 percent of the nation's steel output. The labor system consisted of two types of workers, skilled and unskilled. Skilled workers were highly trained industrial craftsmen who enjoyed high prestige in their communities. They were hired by steel companies under a contract system, and they paid their unskilled helpers out of the lump sums they received from the companies. Variations of this arrangement often existed, in which the steel companies would pay and supply the unskilled workers, who would be supervised by the skilled.

The production of steel was seen as a cooperative endeavor between the company and its skilled labor. These workers were paid a fixed fee per ton of steel produced. The rate fluctuated with the market price of steel, creating in essence a profit-sharing arrangement between the two production partners. Carnegie liked the arrangement. "It is the solution of the capital and labor problem because it really makes them partners—alike in prosperity and adversity" (Stone 1974, 117). Such an arrangement also excluded employers from any control over wages. Once the rate per ton was agreed upon, it was up to the workers to divide the profits.

Craft union control over plant production made it extremely difficult to increase productivity. This situation became particularly important to the companies as the price of steel dropped below the minimum set in contracts with the union. As a result, the cooperative partnership aspect of the contract arrangements disappeared, and companies found themselves paying out an increasing percentage of corporate income to labor. Companies began to recognize that they would have to assert control over production, mechanize operations, and, consequently, break the craft unions. It is interesting to speculate what might have happened had a minimum not been established in the sliding payment scale. The cooperative partnership might have remained intact, the craftspeople would have been forced to accommodate themselves to arrangements that would have assured higher productivity, and the structure of work in the steel industry would probably have evolved quite differently than it did.

The crucial battle for control took place at Carnegie's Homestead Mill in Pittsburgh in 1892. The mill was sealed off with a fence topped by barbed wire, and sentry posts with gun ports were placed along it. Living quarters were built inside for strikebreakers, 300 guards were hired, and the mill was closed. In the following four months, dozens of men were killed in clashes between the workers and guards, scabs, the sheriff, and the Pennsylvania State Militia. The strikers were beaten, and the plant reopened with strikebreakers. Other companies followed suit, and by 1910 the steel industry in the United States was entirely nonunion. Employers were free to mechanize and to restructure the work accordingly. Semiskilled machine operators replaced skilled and unskilled manual laborers. Operations were broken down and simplified to the point where they required neither extensive preparation nor judgment. A new ideology of management and a new set of practitioners had emerged.

The ideal organization was seen as a perfectly rationalized machine—and the manager's role was to create such rationality. Fredrick Taylor, the most influential of these early "management engineers," developed his approach to the organization of work in the steel industry. Taylor's "scientific management" techniques were forerunners of today's industrial engineering and operations research approaches to organizational problems. His emphases on quantification and the use of scientific methods of research and experimentation to maximize efficiency remain basic tenets. Underlying these techniques was the assumption that there should be a clear separation between the persons making decisions about how work should be done and the persons actually doing the work.

The period of rapid technological and managerial innovation ended shortly after 1910, and a comfortable, self-satisfied lethargy settled onto the steel industry. There were few major technological developments or capital investment programs until the 1960s; these programs, partially stimulated by increased foreign competition (Stone 1974), failed to stem the decline that has since brought the domestic steel industry to the brink of extinction. Ironically, a number of plans developed to prevent plants from closing proposed cooperative partnerships between companies and unions, partnerships quite similar to those existing before 1890. In a sense, perhaps, we have come full circle.

There are many parallels between the work force in the steel industry before 1910 and the work force in the health sector after 1910. The bulk of the work force in the health sector in 1910 was physicians, who considered themselves skilled craftspersons. Today physicians compose less than 7 percent of that work force. The preponderance of health workers would probably best be described as semiskilled—they perform fairly narrowly prescribed functions requiring relatively short training periods and usually little judgment. The nature of employment has also changed dramatically. While in 1910 most health workers, including nurses, were self-employed, the vast majority now are salaried employees of an institution. Most radiologists and pathologists still have contract relationships with hospitals (under which they receive a percentage of gross income), and most other physicians remain self-employed fee-for-service practitioners. There has been, however, a gradual shift to group- and salary-based forms of practice. Until the 1960s, while hospitals still enjoyed charitable immunity from malpractice suits, it was not uncommon for surgeons to insist on bringing their own team of nurses to assist them, in much the same way that skilled workers in the steel industry hired their own helpers in the 1890s (Nourian 1978).

The rapid increase in the percentage of the gross national product (GNP) going into the health sector places the modern corporation in a situation not unlike that of the steel companies in 1890, with their fixed payments to craftspersons and declining incomes. While nothing equivalent to the Homestead Steel lockout has taken place with physicians, this similarity has not escaped the notice of many corporations that must pay out an increasing percentage of their income in health benefits for their employees. In every major metropolitan area of this country, business coalitions have been formed to address this problem. One of the solutions currently being examined would assign preferred provider status to providers who offer lower prices. This, in its most uncompromising form, would essentially lock out many physicians and hospitals. (Many younger physicians are already experiencing difficulty obtaining hospital privileges in areas where regional planning controls have restricted the increase in the number of hospital beds.) Taking on the medical societies and the hospital associations today, however, may be more difficult than taking on the Amalgamated Iron, Steel, and Tin Workers was in 1892.

Nursing has been unsuccessful in preventing these changes in working conditions.

The "Proletarianization" of Nursing

In 1910, most Americans were reluctant to enter hospitals for treatment, since most hospitals still carried the stigma of institutions for the destitute. The majority of middle- and upper-class patients received care at home. The private-duty nurse was a major figure in this system of care. Nurses were "trained" in hospital programs, which used these free services to provide much of their nursing care, but almost all nurses then turned to private-duty employment. Most preferred the independence of private-duty nursing, in spite of generally depressed wages, to the substandard pay and working conditions in hospitals.

The Great Depression produced a dramatic shift, however. The difficult economic conditions left many private-duty nurses unemployed. Hospitals survived and were even financially strengthened through the pooled risk schemes of the newly emerging Blue Cross plans. The new hospital insurance programs also stimulated a more rapid replacement of home care by hospital care. The number of salary-based hospital staff nurses as opposed to student nurses grew. Hospitals also created licensed practical nurse programs, one-year technical programs to allow for cheaper labor costs. Taylorism and time and motion studies soon followed, and the pace of nursing in hospitals speeded up. Nurses complained that they were now expected to do in one hour what six nurses had previously done, and many nurses over age 40 began to leave hospital nursing.

Hospitals faced a serious problem in recruiting nurses from the 1940s on. Most continued to prefer the better pay and less factory-like discipline of private-duty nursing. Hospitals resorted to hiring temporary nurses to meet periodic peaks in demand. In many instances, physicians and hospitals controlled private-duty nursing listing services and used this leverage to force nurses to take temporary hospital positions when they were needed. Rapid expansion in the use of hospitals during World War II produced claims of a nursing shortage. This delayed the reduction of shifts to eight hours. Efforts of nurses to increase their salaries were attacked as unpatriotic. The resistance of nurses to employment in hospitals brought threats from President Roosevelt of a nursing draft. The California State Nursing Association, under increasing pressure from its membership, broke from the more submissive past and began to act as the collective bargaining agent for the state's nurses. Other state associations followed suit, largely in an attempt to prevent the encroachment of unionization. Nevertheless, by 1946 private-duty nurses were reduced to a small minority of registered nurses. The freedom to select cases, work independently, provide complete bedside care, and maintain close relationships with physicians and administrators had ended for most nurses (Wagner 1980, 271–90; paraphrased).

The same themes are found in much of the current literature on nursing. Considerable concern is expressed about the supply of nurses. Hospital administration literature devotes much space to strategies for effective recruitment and retention of nurses. Some see changes in working conditions (allowing nurses to do more of the direct patient care that they used to do) rather than higher salary levels as the key to luring back the registered nurses who choose not to work as nurses (Kidder, Gaumer, and Mennemeyer 1981, 105).

Nursing activists have focused their efforts on reestablishing nurses as independent practitioners. A variety of specialized programs has been established to equip nurses for semiautonomous practice. Evaluations of the performance of nurse practitioners giving primary care have concluded that the technical quality of such care is as good as or better than that provided by physicians (for example, Spitzer et al. 1974). Although nurse practitioners generally spend more time with each patient and devote considerably more time to counseling and education, substituting their labor for physicians' could result in cost savings (Spitzer et al. 1974). The critical issue, however, is not establishing the efficiency and efficacy of nurse practitioners, it is determining how they will be paid. Those who control reimbursement will control the destiny of these new practitioners. Current third-party payment policies prohibit direct reimbursement to nurse practitioners. Medicare even prohibits payments (at least on paper) to physicians for the services of nurse practitioners who are not directly supervised by them. Nurse midwives have won the right to bill Pennsylvania Blue Shield directly for their services, and there have been breakthroughs in other states. It is not clear, however, whether nurse practitioners will ever gain a strong foothold as independent providers (at least for billing purposes); like nurses in the 1930s, they may simply be absorbed by medical practices and hospitals as a means of increasing productivity and income. The rise in malpractice insurance costs for such providers, however, has raised a new barrier to their use either as independent or physician-affiliated practitioners.

These developments are overshadowed by the exponential growth in both numbers and types of allied health personnel. These individuals find employment almost exclusively in institutional settings. All have attempted to move toward professionalization, as nurses did, and to a large extent have met barriers. Just as the iron- and steelworkers' guilds frustrated the steel companies by resisting technological innovation, more rational task allocation, and more economical service provision, so the newly licensed technicians and aspiring health professionals frustrate hospital boards and administrators. Efforts have been made to resist the licensure of any new allied health occupation, and proposals to create institutional licensure instead of the current fragmented, individual licensure programs are generated periodically. Should such a proposal succeed, it would achieve essentially what the lockout achieved at Homestead Mill and greatly enhance the flexibility of institutions to organize the work that goes on within them. Health care facilities, for better or worse, could then truly enter the industrial era. The industrial sector appears to be moving in the opposite direction—toward recovering some of its earlier sense of common purpose. American corporations, faced with increasing competition from Japanese corporations, are attempting to learn quickly from their rivals, whose paternalistic commitment to their work force (and the resulting institutional loyalty) creates an environment similar to that found in many American hospitals.

SUMMARY AND CONCLUSIONS

The construction of our current health system has taken more than 80 years. Unlike a building, whose construction is guided by blueprints, it has evolved in response to conflicting cultural pressures, more like a geological formation. Those pressures—to define health care as an economic good, as a social relationship, and as a professional service— have produced four basic structural changes.

Size

Not only does the health care system now absorb almost three times as much of a substantially increased GNP as it used to, its scale of operations has grown significantly. The average size of acute-care hospitals has more than doubled in the last 30 years, while acute-care hospitals with fewer than 50 beds have all but disappeared. Nursing homes have witnessed a similar increase in average size since 1965, and Medicare safety requirements have essentially eliminated the converted wood frame houses that provided residents smaller, often more home-like environments; some argue that more was lost than gained thereby. Physicians, formerly staunch entrepreneurs, have increasingly chosen to practice in group and corporation-like settings, such as some of the larger HMOs.

Specialization

At the turn of the century, 90 percent of all health workers were physicians, and as many as 90 percent of these physicians were general practitioners. Today, physicians account for less than 7 percent of all health workers, and little more than 10 percent of them identify themselves as general practitioners. More than 30 different health professionals and allied health professionals receive licensing from state boards.

At the same time that a highly complex division of labor was emerging among health care workers, shifts were taking place among facilities. At the turn of the century, hospitals cared for the destitute and homeless, the chronically ill, and the acutely ill. Later, boarding and nursing homes absorbed the first two responsibilities, and acute-care hospitals began to specialize even further in terms of the services they would provide. Many, because of financial exigencies, have begun to back away from providing a full range of services.

Centralization

Not only are services now provided in larger, more specialized settings, but these settings are increasingly linked together into more centralized systems of services. Over one-third of all U.S. community hospitals are now part of multihospital systems, and this number appears to be growing at the rate of 3 percent a year (Ermann and Gabel 1984, 52). While accurate figures for ambulatory services are more difficult to come by, it appears that an increasing proportion of local HMOs has been absorbed into larger voluntary and insurance company–sponsored systems. The proportion of freestanding facilities for long-term care is substantially lower, and the growth of multi-institutional systems for long-term care has been substantially more rapid in recent years than has the growth of acute-care hospital systems.

Privatization

Until the passage of Medicare and Medicaid in 1965, private providers of services were much like solo fee-for-service physicians—essentially small-scale owner-operated entrepreneurial ventures. Private hospitals were predominantly locally owned, physician-owned, located in the South and Southwest, and constructed in communities lacking voluntary facilities. Privately owned facilities for long-term care were almost exclusively owner operated, many being simply converted residences developed in response to restrictions on eligibility for old-age assistance to institutionalized persons (in voluntary and public facilities) in the 1934 Social Security legislation. Investor-owned multi-institutional systems have grown dramatically since 1965. In contrast to not-for-profit multihospital systems, for-profit systems tend to be larger (averaging 23 hospitals per system as opposed to 7) and more geographically dispersed (located in several states). Investor-owned systems have also moved far more rapidly into the acquisition of freestanding nursing homes and psychiatric hospitals (Ermann and Gabel 1984, 54). With the passage of Medicare, investments in health care might produce large profits rather than losses. In fact, health care became the hottest investment area on the stock market. The definition of health care as an economic good rather than a social relationship or professional service gained ascendency. The formula for the development of all these new investor-owned systems was (1) study the Medicare legislation and regulations, (2) form a corporation, (3) go public to raise capital, (4) acquire more and more health care facilities, and (5) make a profit for all concerned (Wohl 1984). The profits attracted investors such as Standard Oil and Dow Chemical, assuring a degree of stability in the corporate hospital sector. This was followed by branching out into emergicenters, surgicenters, and other forms of delivery.

The larger new hospital corporations are now in a position to consider prestige and visibility when buying facilities. In 1983, for example, Hospital Corporation of America entered into negotiations with Massachusetts General Hospital to purchase McLean Psychiatric Hospital, which is affiliated with the Harvard medical school. These negotiations are stalled because of resistance from the McLean medical staff and the dean's advisory committee, but they are likely to be successful eventually. American Medical International is trying to lease or buy the hospital center of George Washington University.

Why did these structural shifts take place? Are they the result of powerful, inevitable forces that it would be a sheer waste of energy to oppose? Will the health care system continue to consolidate into larger, more specialized, more centralized, and more privately owned systems of delivery, or will the contradictions of such developments catch up with it and push it in the opposite direction? In the next chapter we will describe the mechanics of the existing system, and in the final chapter of this section we will begin to assess the relative contribution of these structural shifts to the performance of the system. We will then be in a position to explore in more detail the choices for survival in the labyrinth.

2

Blueprints

Two hospital administrators on a camping trip in the Rocky Mountains wake up in the middle of the night, hearing a grizzly bear prowling around outside their tent. One rushes to pull on his jogging shoes. Puzzled, the other asks, "George, what are you doing? There's no way we can outrun that bear, we've got to think through a different plan." George stares back and says with gritted teeth, "I don't have to outrun that bear, all I have to do is outrun you."

Perhaps more than ever before, medical groups, hospitals, and other providers are staring at each other with gritted teeth, like our "friend" George. They are trying to calculate their relative strengths and weaknesses in order to assess their prospects for survival in an environment of increasingly scarce resources and increasingly stiff competition. Many health care providers are going through exercises similar to those at Fleet Foot Hospital.

Fleet Foot Hospital

George stared with a growing sense of uneasiness at the numbers the hospital's planner had pulled together the previous evening. Earlier projections of an increase in admissions seemed off target. While occupancy levels had climbed steadily, in spite of a declining length of stay since 1980, there was a sudden drop of 10 percent in average occupancy in 1985. What was happening?

Market share had not changed: Fleet Foot had maintained its 31 percent share of the acute-care patient-days in the Block Grant metropolitan area. The slight drop in overall population could not explain the drop in admissions, because the population of the metropolitan area was generally aging.

A number of changes had taken place, however. The prospective payment system had been put in place in the state for Medicare and Medicaid; it provided adjusted-case (rather than per diem, cost-related) reimbursement. Several HMOs had been aggressively marketing in their service area. The projected shifts toward an older population had been used to justify a substantial increase in the number of skilled nursing home beds in the metropolitan area, as well as expanded support for home care programs. Further, as a result of a recent collective bargaining agreement, one of the major employers had traded wage increases for major reductions in benefits, including a substantial, new coinsurance and deductible provision in the company's hospital insurance plan. The number of specialty and multispecialty groups in the region had grown, and some had hired full-time professional managers. Some of these acquired the ability to perform complex diagnostic and laboratory procedures, and one had been exploring the feasibility of developing a freestanding surgicenter.

Fleet Foot may not know it yet, but there is a grizzly bear outside its tent as well. In order to fully grasp the implications of this situation, one must understand the pathways of the health system as a whole. In this chapter, therefore, we focus on mapping relationships among significant components of the system. After we have completed this review of the dynamics of the system, we will look at the choices available to Fleet Foot Hospital.

HEALTH SERVICES AS AN OPEN SYSTEM

Figure 2.1 presents the health services as an open system, a concept borrowed from early computer systems theory and one as applicable to biological organisms as it is to social structures (Katz and Kahn 1978). It enables us to view the health system as a dynamic, living organism interacting with a larger environment.

Any open system must take energy from its environment. This energy is derived from raw materials (patients), manpower (physicians and others), technology (drugs, mechanical devices, knowledge), and money. The system must combine these inputs into throughputs (for example, treatments or therapies) that will lead eventually to certain outputs (health, death, profit, loss, morale, staff turnover, and so on). These outputs are processed in some way by the environment, which

Figure 2.1 An Open System

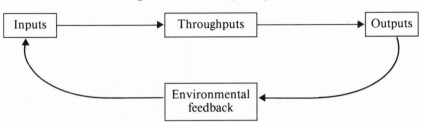

may produce new inputs (such as indignant letters, malpractice suits, satisfied repeat customers, and more or fewer financial resources). The system then adapts to these new or changed inputs. Adaptation often becomes routine, a series of standard operating or coping procedures that attempts, almost automatically, to adjust the system. This adaptive mechanism operates as a thermostat, attempting to maintain a dynamic homeostasis while at the same time attempting to preserve the basic character of the system. For example, more or fewer workers are re-cruited and more or fewer hospital beds created, presumably in re-sponse to changing environmental needs. Further, as illustrated in chap-ter 1, all open systems have a tendency to move toward greater complexity.

An open system can be broken down into five components, or subsystems (Katz and Kahn 1978), each of which plays an essential role in assuring the survival of the whole. These components include those individuals, departments, and institutions performing the following tasks: (1) production, (2) support, (3) maintenance, (4) adaptation, and (5) management of the system. The major inputs, throughputs, and out-puts of each of these components as they occur in the health system are summarized in figure 2.2.

The *production component* consists of all the primary providers in the health system—hospitals, nursing homes, outpatient clinics, physi-cians, and health departments. These institutions and individuals are directly involved in processing the raw material, that is, the patients. Like the production department in an industrial plant, this direct care component tends to have a more highly developed, specialized, and standardized technology than the other components.

The *support component* procures needed inputs and disposes of the larger system's outputs. Its purpose is to secure maximum control over the environment. Third-party payment mechanisms provide the needed financial resources; professional associations lobby for support within the political arena; public relations efforts of hospitals and com-

Figure 2.2 Functional Components of the Health Care System

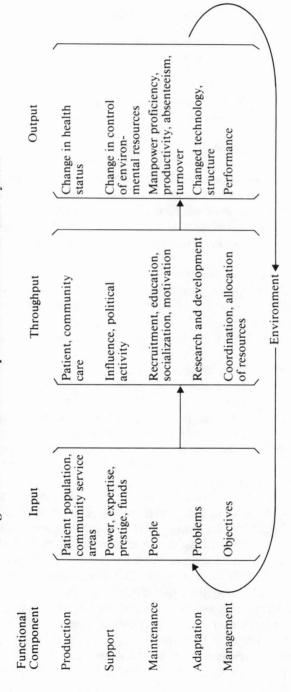

Functional Component	Input	Throughput	Output
Production	Patient population, community service areas	Patient, community care	Change in health status
Support	Power, expertise, prestige, funds	Influence, political activity	Change in control of environmental resources
Maintenance	People	Recruitment, education, socialization, motivation	Manpower proficiency, productivity, absenteeism, turnover
Adaptation	Problems	Research and development	Changed technology, structure
Management	Objectives	Coordination, allocation of resources	Performance

Environment

munity agencies attempt to assure a supply of consumers. Until recently, the health system has been quite successful in getting what it wanted from the larger society—in other words, the support component has been very effective.

The *maintenance component* is concerned with the upkeep of the equipment, both physical and human, involved in production. Major emphasis is placed on sustaining the skill, motivation, morale, and, consequently, the effectiveness of the work force. Educational programs attempt to shape individuals to fit roles within the system, and personnel departments become involved with on-the-job training and job redesign in order to achieve desired levels of effectiveness. As we explained in chapter 1, the health system is itself part of society's maintenance component, and this accounts for some of its distinctive character.

The *adaptation component* attempts to assure the system's survival within a changing environment. Periodic adjustments are required by scientific advances, changes in public expectations, and shifting disease patterns within the population. Adaptive elements such as medical schools and other research centers have supplied a complex, ever-expanding array of technological procedures for dealing with specific medical problems. Little has been done, however, to address the organizational implications of these technological changes. It is ironic that the existing, although limited, efforts, particularly at the federal level (for example, the National Center for Health Services Research and Technology Assessment and the Health Care Financing Administration's Office of Research, Demonstrations, and Statistics), have received a disproportionate share of recent budget cuts.

The *managerial component* coordinates and directs the activities of the other components. This has been and remains by far the most underdeveloped component of the health system. Existing structures (health systems agencies, state hospital rate-setting commissions, and so on) focus on controlling only a narrow aspect of the activities of the overall system. Until recently, enough resources were poured into the health system to allow most of its components to expand and develop. The flow of dollars was sufficiently unrestricted that one component could make gains without jeopardizing the gains of the other components. As a result, the more rigorous resource-allocation decisions, commonly associated with a well-developed formalized managerial component (or an effectively functioning competitive market), were unnecessary. The informal managerial mechanisms were adequate, and the more formal ones, such as planning agencies, appear to have been used largely as window dressing. It now seems that this period of rapid and easy growth is over. It appears that the upper limits of the resources that society is willing to allocate without any additional growth in personal income have been reached (Getzen 1984). When there are no longer sufficient resources to satisfy the appetites of the major health constituencies, differences in objectives will be brought into sharper focus, and the need for formal managerial controls (or their counterparts in the competitive market) will become obvious.

We are currently witnessing a struggle for control of the formal managerial component that is emerging in the health sector. The American Medical Association, the American Hospital Association, medical schools, planning agencies, third parties, investor-owned multi-institutional systems, federal agencies, and private non-health-related corporations (the major purchasers of health services, through the insurance benefits they provide their employees) are battling to determine who will coordinate and, therefore, control the system. The focus of this confrontation will change as various schemes for the reorganization and financing of care are proposed. No matter whether such controls are more competitive or regulatory in orientation, how they are shaped will affect both how the objectives of the system and of health care itself are defined and whose interests those controls will serve.

THE CONTROL GATEWAYS

Figure 2.3 shows the relationships among the various components in more detail. There are five key locations within the health system where the managerial component, no matter who controls it, can operate gateways to shape the outputs of the system. The mechanics of the gateways are not well understood, and so far the operation of them has been uncoordinated. We will discuss each of the gateways briefly before deciding how Fleet Foot Hospital can deal with the problems it faces. Each gateway involves the use of money to shape the output of the system. Only by following the money can one make sense of the outputs.

Gateway 1: Translating Need into Demand

A population's demographic characteristics will generate an array of health care needs, as defined by providers of services and the population itself. These needs will be related to (1) the prevention of disease and the promotion of health, (2) the care of persons with short-term illnesses, and (3) the maintenance of persons with chronic diseases and disabilities. The translation of these needs into demand depends on the willingness of those individuals and families with such needs to seek

Figure 2.3   Five Management Control Gateways in the Health Care System

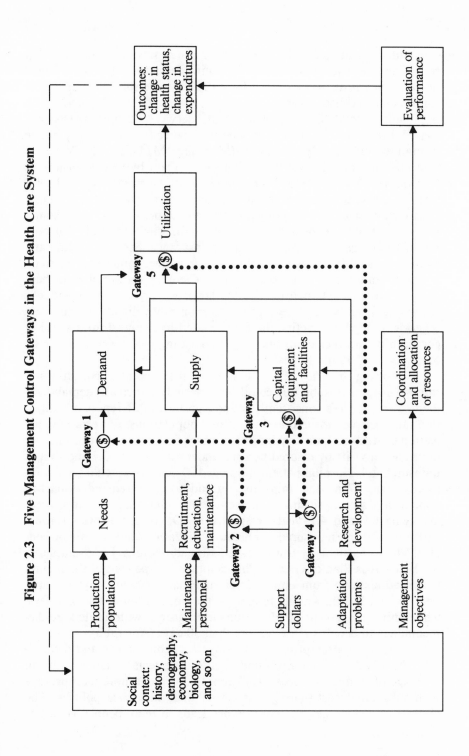

care and the willingness of those supplying such services to provide that care. The ease with which needs flow into demand is affected by how much money is available (in the form of insurance subsidies) and what controls are exercised over it.

Only a small fraction of all health services (20 percent) is purchased directly by the consumer. About 40 percent is covered by public insurance and subsidy programs (Medicare, Medicaid, the Veterans Administration, and so on) and about 40 percent by private insurance (Carroll and Arnett 1981). There are several major reasons that health care has been so insulated from the forces of the marketplace. First, health care involves unevenly distributed, unpredictable, and sometimes catastrophic expenditures that the individual can deal with only through pooling risks—that is, through insurance. Second, health care, as we suggested in chapter 1, occupies a grey area, somewhere between a private commodity and a public good. There are certain obvious benefits, or positive externalities, for the larger society in the individual's remaining healthy and free from communicable diseases. There are other, less tangible benefits; these are related to the need for a sense of community and the revulsion toward allocating health services strictly on the basis of ability to pay.

Lowering the price of health services at the point of consumption through insurance subsidies could be expected to increase demand for them. Surveys have consistently found significant differences in utilization rates between insured and uninsured populations. For example, the National Medical Care Expenditure survey found the average number of physician visits by insured persons under age 65 to be 3.7 and that of uninsured 2.4. Hospital patient-days per 100 persons were 90 for the insured versus 47 for the uninsured. In addition, insured individuals in poor health see physicians 70 percent more often than the uninsured, averaging 6.9 and 4.1 visits, respectively (Davis and Rowland 1983, 160–65). Within the insured population, utilization tends to mirror benefits. This is particularly true of psychiatric admissions. For example, in the Blue Cross Plan of Greater Philadelphia, 44.4 percent of the mental health admissions from employer groups that offer 365 days of inpatient mental health benefits remain in the hospital more than 30 days, while only 16.5 percent of admissions from groups with limited, 30-day mental health benefits remain more than 30 days (Apt 1983).

In a major attempt to test the impact of coinsurance and deductibles, the Rand Corporation found significant effects. Persons with full coverage of medical services spend about 50 percent more than persons with substantial cost-sharing features in their insurance policies. The absence of deductibles and coinsurance leads to more people using services and to more services being used per user. Use of ambulatory services and hospital admissions was a third higher among individuals with full coverage, however the use of services did not differ once patients were admitted to the hospital (Newhouse et al. 1981, Brook, Ware, and Rogers 1983).

Most proposals for more competition have focused on this particular gateway. Enthoven has argued for a limit on the tax-exempt status of employee benefit packages, because, he argues, they have artificially stimulated demand for health insurance coverage (Enthoven 1978). Blue Cross plans, long proponents of full-service benefits for hospital care, have introduced provisions for coinsurance and deductibles in an effort to control costs and keep their premiums competitive. This approach has been advocated by many who believe that increasing the consumer's sensitivity to price is the only way to control utilization and, thus, costs of health insurance programs.

A variation of this approach, the preferred provider organization, uses higher coinsurance and deductibles to steer subscribers away from more expensive providers. Since a routine obstetric stay, for example, may cost three times as much at one hospital as at another, such disincentives can produce significant savings for the plan. Some Blue Cross plans, following the lead of more aggressive HMOs, are offering cash bonuses to subscribers for early discharge in routine obstetric admissions. Eliminating the financial incentives of hospital insurance programs that stimulate the substitution of less costly outpatient services for inpatient ones has long been an argument in support of the development of HMOs.

The kinds of controls or red tape involved in the use of services can also reduce utilization and produce savings. Increasing attention has been given, for example, to the use of mandatory second opinions to curb unnecessary surgery. Available evidence suggests that mandatory second opinions probably save more money than they cost. For example, 16 percent of individuals in New York City who were required by their insurance companies to obtain second opinions failed to have their initial diagnosis confirmed (Ruchlin, Finkel, and McCarthy 1982). Similarly, review of the mandatory second-opinion program that is required by the Massachusetts Medicaid program found that 14.5 percent of recommended surgical procedures were not confirmed by the second opinion (Martin et al. 1982). Peer Review Organizations, which are responsible for reviewing admissions and procedures for Medicare payment, have been given broad powers to restrict certification for payment. This potential has been viewed with increasing concern by providers.

Gateway 2: Adjusting the Supply of Health Manpower

The second gateway can expand or contract the overall supply of personnel, and it can alter the mix of personnel. In the last 20 years, federal subsidies have expanded the number of physicians produced by medical schools. There is little agreement, however, on the impact this will have. Conventional economic wisdom suggests that, if you increase the supply of physicians, you will decrease the unit cost of physician services through competition, but there is no clear evidence that this is happening. Historically, low physician-to-population ratios have been positively related to physician fees, suggesting that physicians tend to create their own prices depending on what income they desire (Reinhardt 1984). They achieve their target incomes in part by adjusting fees and in part by providing more elaborate services (performing more tests, procedures, and so on per patient visit; requiring more extensive follow-up visits; and so forth). There is also a tendency for physicians to practice regardless of the volume of need they confront; the oversupply of physicians combined with insured services, may induce demand.

Surgical rates differ strikingly among areas of the country and are highly correlated with surgeon-to-population ratios. Projections of existing surgical rates suggest that over 70 percent of the women in one city in Maine will have had their uterus removed by the time they reach 75, while in another city only 20 miles away only 25 percent will have had their uterus removed by age 75 (Wennberg and Gittelsohn 1982, 120).

Conventional economic wisdom might also suggest that the production of less expensive substitutes would produce savings, however such physician "extenders" tend to supplement rather than substitute for physicians' services. A nurse practitioner may be able to handle 70 percent of the services provided by a primary care physician, thus reducing the unit cost for these services by 50 percent. The same primary care physician, however, now supervising four nurse practitioners, can generate four times the services at three times the cost. As a result, third parties may be charged as much as four times more for the services provided by that physician's office. These multiplier effects have been so staggering that most third parties have refused all but the most restrictive payments for the services of these new practitioners, thus undermining the intent of federal support for the development of these programs as a means of increasing primary care in underserved areas.

The conventional economic wisdom regarding supply appears to work in the case of registered nurses. In contrast to physicians, nurses are almost exclusively salaried employees and generate little demand for additional service. Most hospitals attempt to control, informally or formally, the wages of nurses in their area. In the case of nursing, stimulation of additional supply would appear to assist in controlling labor costs, whereas a decreased pool would force regional salary increases and greater attention to working conditions.

Gateway 3: Adjusting Capital Expenditures

Capital equipment, unlike labor, utilities, or disposable supplies, is not consumed in the year it is purchased. Capital expenditures, therefore, have far longer lasting consequences on operating costs, overall capacity, and the character of the system. As a result, they tend to be controlled, budgeted, and paid for quite differently from operating expenses.

The assumption that utilization will expand to meet the capacity available has long been a part of the conventional wisdom of the health sector.

> *Shain and Roemer's Law:*
> *A Bed Built Is a Bed Filled*
>
> It is an obvious but often overlooked fact that, once hospital beds are built, they tend to be used. Total costs for hospital care in a community will be directly related to the number of beds available in that community. To illustrate this rule, Shain and Roemer (1959) looked at the bed supply in every county in upstate New York and in every state in the union. They found a high correlation between hospital days per thousand persons and beds per thousand persons. More than 70 percent of the differences in hospital use was related to differences in supply. Common sense would argue that, in those communities with fewer beds, occupancy rates would be higher. Even when deviation from expected occupancy (given the size of the facilities in question) is taken into account in comparing the upstate New York counties, less than 25 percent of the variation is accounted for by the number of beds per thousand persons. In short, "within units common to the United States, general hospital beds are occupied at about the same rate, regardless of whether there are few or many beds per thousand population" (Shain and Roemer 1959, 73).

A more recent and precise estimate of this effect on use suggests that a 10 percent decrease in the number of hospital beds would produce about a 4 percent decrease in bed-days among Medicare beneficiaries (Ginzberg and Koretz 1983).

This corollary of Parkinson's law applies not just to beds, but to almost every piece of capital equipment purchased. New equipment such as the lithotriptor and magnetic resonance imaging have made possible rapid, noninvasive diagnosis and treatment. Just as the Xerox copier has affected the written documentation produced by bureaucracy and business, so this new technology has produced a geometric proliferation of diagnostic procedures in hospitals and physicians' offices. When the capacity of existing facilities and equipment is expanded, it is used.

This awareness has spawned three generations of efforts to control capital expenditures and appears to be on its way to spawning a fourth. The precursors of the current health planning agencies were voluntary community groups established in the 1940s and 1950s by local business leaders. At that time, local philanthropy was a critical component in the financing of capital improvements. The passage of Medicare and Medicaid in 1965 enabled hospitals to enter the capital markets with much the same status as public utilities. By 1979 debt financing of short-term hospital construction accounted for over 70 percent of capital expenditures ("Hospital Indicators" 1981). Third parties have supported this debt financing by reimbursing hospitals for their interest payments and depreciation. While Medicare and Medicaid reimbursement of capital costs under state certificate-of-need laws takes place only with approval, there is little other control over reimbursement. Decisions are made autonomously, with little pooled information, and they are often based on quite different criteria. Indeed, by not requiring hospitals to fund depreciation of their capital equipment and improvements, the existing mechanism for reimbursing capital costs has actually spurred facilities into shortsighted expansion. Since interest costs and depreciation are generally reimbursed by third parties, and since these payments exceed debt payments in the first few years, the facility gains a short-term windfall. Later shortfalls, resulting from declining interest payments as a proportion of overall debt payments, create pressure for further capital expansion. There are now efforts to change the way hospitals are paid for capital costs. The current approach is carried to its logical absurdity in the following account:

The Tale of Stephen O'Toole

O'Toole, an enterprising hospital accountant, undertakes to persuade a wealthy, dying dowager to donate money for a hospital wing, instead of giving her estate to Ralph Nader to eliminate slums and unemployment. Five to ten percent upfront money is all that's needed to begin a construction boom that will solve the problems that concern her. Having explained the income that can be generated by third-party payment of interest expenses and depreciation, he launches into his final sales pitch:

"Now let me go on," said the young man. "Perhaps you can see how these things overlap. The extra cash you generate in a new building helps to pay the cash shortage on the building which is ten years old. And the extra depreciation payments on a building twenty years old make up any difference. Take my word for it, the best way to arrange the finances of a hospital is to build it in a series of seven pavilions, one every five years."

"Well," said Mrs. O'Leary, "I'm sure that's all very clever and important. But I don't really see it as a way to clear slums, whereas Mr. Nader . . ."

"Please forgive me for interrupting," said O'Toole, "but there is a point I haven't mentioned. You will notice that the seven-pavilion system assumes that you will tear down the oldest pavilion in order to make room for the new one. But a forty-year-old hospital is still a useful building, even if it is all paid up.

"My proposal is that we just let it stand and keep on building pavilions at a rate that will accelerate as the depreciation starts rolling in. I calculate that you could convert all the slums of Chicago into hospital pavilions in another fifty years after you got rolling."

Mrs. O'Leary pondered, then asked, "But where would all those people live?"

"Very simple. They would become hospital employees. That solves the unemployment problem too. You may wonder whether there would be enough patients to fill all the beds, but that can be accomplished by increasing the ratio of employees to patients. At the present time the average is four employees per patient, but it is growing fast. There are already two local hospitals with a ratio of 7.5 to 1; and it only needs to reach 100 to 1 to take care of the patient shortage."

"Whatever the ratio is in this hospital right now," the lady tartly remarked, "it isn't enough to get someone to answer the buzzer."

"You see what I mean," grinned O'Toole.

"Yes, I do. Call my lawyer, young man. I'm going to write a will" (Fisher 1980, 5–8).

Health systems agencies, the current vehicle for controlling the likes of Mr. O'Toole, have faced much criticism and, possibly, fatal federal budgetary disfavor. In order for new facilities or equipment above a certain cost to be reimbursed by Medicare and Medicaid, hospitals must receive a certificate of need from the state. The review process required for a certificate of need involves, at least from the perspective of a facility administrator, massive documentation and interminable reviews at the local, area, and state levels. Without a certificate of need, however, a facility will not be able to borrow money from major lenders and will, barring a very healthy private endowment to subsidize its ventures, be stalemated. "The certificate-of-need law will," one lawyer announced excitedly at a public discussion after the state passed certificate-of-need legislation in Pennsylvania, "assure the full employment of the legal profession in the way that Medicare cost reimbursement requirements assured full employment of accountants!" That prediction has proved largely accurate, and health systems agency staff, embroiled in this adversary situation, have had little time to make the certificate-of-need process more coherent through systematic regional planning. Facility associations have complained about the costs of the process and the delays it creates, which produce even more increases in project costs because of inflation in the construction industry. In terms of overall health system costs, pushing all of these projects and their resulting capital and operating costs farther downstream has probably produced significant savings, although nobody, at least publicly, is making such an argument. It is hard to view inertia as a form of efficiency.

Health Systems Agencies
in Memoriam

In planning, the theory is to be regional,
Though in practice, this is seasonal.

In theory, one must skim the cream,
And leave health care trim and lean.

The practice is delusional,
Making the sane seclusional.

Yet, HSAs were never meant to stay,
Like old soldiers, they'll just fade away.

When the new battles become clear,
We may wish they still were here.

Clearly, controlling units of service has proved an extremely cumbersome way to control capital expenditures and their resulting impact on operating costs. An assessment of the impact of state certificate-of-need controls between 1966 and 1972 concluded that, while these controls slowed the rate of growth of hospital bed supply, they tended to increase the investment in quality-enhancing projects. The overall outcome was that, while hospital days per thousand were slightly reduced by certificates of need, the cost per day increased, producing essentially no impact on overall costs (Salkever and Bice 1976, 204).

Some states have attempted to exercise greater control over actual expenditures. New York, for example, attempted to develop a capital expenditure budget in much the way that individual institutions do, requiring that individual certificate-of-need proposals be batched and that an overall budgetary limit be maintained. New Jersey has attempted to establish the principle that third-party-funded depreciation is a pooled regional fund not owned by any individual institution. The next generation of health planning agencies will no doubt attempt to reestablish the link between the third parties that are paying for capital expenditures and those who plan such expenditures, a link that was lost in the transformation of early local philanthropic and business prototypes to community health planning agencies and, subsequently, health systems agencies.

Gateway 4: Adjusting Research and Development

The research and development subsystem, much like the support subsystem, acts as an energy booster, raising the voltage or pressure in other parts of the system by (1) creating demand for new services, (2) generating pressure for an increasingly well trained work force, and (3) increasing pressures for new capital expenditures. The ethical necessity for using existing knowledge to improve health and cure disease infuses the system with new energy. The overall pace of such scientific and technological developments can be slowed down or speeded up, however, by increasing support for research and development or shifting the emphasis of this support. One might, for example, increasingly focus support on those research and development activities that are less costly or that may result in cost savings for the system. It is not always possible, however, to predict such outcomes in advance.

The rapidity with which these innovations are implemented is affected by the support provided for them at gateways 1, 2, and 3. It is also affected by the ease with which they can be utilized and paid for in clinical settings. New drugs, for example, which must be approved by the Food and Drug Administration before they can be used, generally require far greater documentation and review than do plans for new facilities, which must undergo the certificate-of-need process. The willingness with which third parties reimburse these new procedures facilitates their development and adoption. Since most health insurance policies in the past made little distinction between experimental and standard therapies, new technologies such as the coronary bypass operation and hip replacement became increasingly sophisticated and were made increasingly available to the population (Bunker, Fowles, and Schaffarzick 1982).

Gateway 5: Adjusting the Production of Services

The fifth pressure point, and the one most commonly associated with the managerial function, involves the production of services—the pairing of supply and demand to produce utilization. We know far more about how to work this gateway than the others. Decisions concerning the coordination and allocation of resources at the point of delivery affect the cost, number, and nature of the products produced, as well as their subsequent impact on the health of the population. These decisions are not unlike those facing the restaurateur, who must decide the quality and mix of ingredients, the recipes, and the setting in which they will be served. Those decisions will be affected by what the restaurant is expected to serve, the fixed and variable costs associated with its operation, and whatever special payment arrangements and discounts the restaurateur has worked out with potential customers to attract their patronage.

If we are going to imagine the health care provider as a restaurateur, it may be useful to imagine the consumer as a college freshman, away from home for the first time and with a very large appetite. This particular freshman is fortunate: he has a rich and indulgent uncle. "Give my nephew the very best and I'll pay whatever the reasonable costs are—as long as I'm fairly certain that you're not padding the bill," says the uncle. This is, in essence, cost-based reimbursement, as it was adopted after World War II by Blue Cross plans and later by Medicare and Medicaid as a means for paying hospitals. A patron like this freshman is a lot of fun to provide services for: the restaurateur does not have to worry about the cost of ingredients and is free to create culinary masterpieces. Hospitals under cost-based reimbursement responded likewise and, as will be described in more detail in the next chapter, costs increased rapidly.

The restaurant at which the rich uncle treated, however, was in the city. Our college freshman had to get most of his meals in the fast-food shops (outpatient clinics, physicians' offices) surrounding the campus. Since this nephew came from the poor side of the family (eligible for Medicaid), the uncle agreed to pay a fixed sum for every meal these fast-food restaurants served his nephew. This fixed amount, however, was usually quite a bit less than what it actually cost to provide the meals. As a result, fewer of the fast-food restaurants in the campus area were willing to provide meals for the nephew; of those that did, some tried to trick the uncle by double billing (fraud) or by serving breakfast, lunch, dinner, and a midnight snack all at the same sitting ("pingpong-ing," a form of abuse that involves performing multiple and usually unnecessary procedures and tests in a single office visit). Predictably, many local restaurants would encourage the nephew, when he showed up looking hungry, to go to the big restaurant in the metropolis (in which they had an interest), where the uncle would pick up the actual tab. (Not surprisingly, persons with Medicaid tend to be treated more often in acute-care hospitals than in outpatient facilities, in situations where outpatient services can adequately substitute for inpatient ser-vices.)

This particular college freshman was not the only one who had a rich uncle. The other students' rich uncles, however, had not bothered with the kind of arrangement that the first uncle had developed with the restaurant in the metropolis. In their case, any restaurant could sim-ply send their uncles the bill for the meal and the uncles would pay it. Although these charges were higher than the restaurants' costs, the un-cles did not have to deal with all the details of restaurant operation. Even though the first uncle got a discount from the city restaurant, the restaurant benefited from the uncle's rapid, predictable payment. (This is, in essence, the rationale for the Blue Cross "discount," which in-volves paying on a daily or weekly basis the estimated average costs per day for Blue Cross subscribers being treated and then making a year-end settlement based on what those average costs actually were.) The first uncle, being a shrewd businessman, refused to pay any costs that were not directly associated with providing meals for his nephew. He refused, for example, to pay any portion of the costs associated with customers whose checks bounced or who disappeared before the coffee was served. Eventually the discrepancy between allowable costs and ac-tual costs grew. This particular uncle fell on hard times and tried to economize by disallowing more costs. He even attempted to impose budgets on the meals served by the city restaurant ahead of time so that he could make these expenditures more predictable and control any increase in them. (For hospitals, the equivalent is prospective reimbursement.) What could the poor restaurateur do but attempt to recover his losses by shifting them onto the bills of those who paid the actual prices (or charges) on the menu? For those restaurants in which the bulk of the customers paid charges, this was relatively easy to do. However, for those restaurants in which most of the customers had, through their uncles, worked out an arrangement to pay only allowable costs, this was far more difficult to do.

How could the latter restaurants possibly survive, to say nothing of competing with those restaurants supported by the rich uncles who paid the prices on the menu? They were actually losing money on each meal served and sliding slowly into bankruptcy. There were screams of outrage from the uncles who were paying the actual prices, or charges. Why should they be forced to subsidize those uncles who paid less than the actual costs of the meals? In those areas of the country where the differentials were too great, such as the Northeast, the uncles just moved their business elsewhere. "There are plenty of good universities and restaurants in the Southwest, and everybody there pays the charges," they reasoned (just as many commercial insurance companies have all but conceded the market in the Northeast to the Blues and Medicare and Medicaid). That, however, did not do much for the financial viability of the restaurants (hospitals) in the Northeast.

The rhetoric and lobbying became intense. One alternative suggested was to develop an equitable price that all of the uncles would pay, some kind of uniform prospective charge that would take into account the fact that it is usually cheaper to provide breakfast than dinner just as an appendectomy is usually cheaper than coronary bypass surgery. Reimbursing hospitals on the basis of length of stay is like reimbursing restaurants for the amount of time that a table is occupied rather than what is served. This is, in effect, the way hospitals have been traditionally reimbursed. Not surprisingly, payers have found service a bit slow and have imposed all kinds of relatively ineffective utilization review controls. Reimbursement on the basis of DRGs, a system of prospective reimbursement developed in New Jersey and implemented nationally by Medicare, attempts to eliminate this particular perversity by paying a fixed price, in line with regional averages, for a particular illness. Not surprisingly, average length of stay in New Jersey hospitals dropped significantly, and similar results are now taking place nationwide.

These schemes do not do away with all of the irrational utilization incentives of the fast-food restaurants (outpatient facilities) and the city restaurant (hospital). Why not set a fixed price for all food provided to a student? The restaurateur would then have an incentive to economize and, quite possibly, to give the student a better overall deal for his uncle's money. The restaurateur would be creating a dormitory food service plan (in the health care context, a capitation system, or HMO). Let us look at how the management component of an HMO might work.

OPERATING THE GATEWAYS:
THE CASE OF THE HMO

Many HMOs, unlike conventional hospitals or office practices, have effectively manipulated all five of the managerial control gateways we have described. Let us look at how each of these gateways might be operated within such a delivery system.

Gateway 1: Translating Need into Demand in an HMO

The key to the success of HMOs has been their significantly lower hospitalization experience when contrasted with conventional insurance plans (Luft 1981). With hospital days per thousand as much as 40 percent below that of conventional hospital insurance plans, they are able to offer a comprehensive package of benefits at little more than, and sometimes less than, the premium for conventional plans. Although nobody is quite sure how gateway 1 works in HMOs, it appears to result from a conscious strategy to (1) avoid adverse risk selection and (2) use financial incentives to assure lower inpatient utilization.

At first glance, HMOs might appear prone to adverse risk selection, since the more comprehensive benefits they offer would substantially lower the anticipated out-of-pocket costs of an illness-prone individual eligible for such a plan. Actually, patients who see a physician frequently and are consequently more likely to be a higher risk form bonds with their physician and are reluctant to sever them in order to join a new form of practice. Individuals with weak or nonexistent ties to practitioners (probably younger and certainly healthier) are more likely to join an HMO. Particularly important for an HMO in avoiding adverse risk selection is the out-of-pocket price of its premiums relative to the other options available to potential subscribers through their employee benefits plans. Who would enroll in a special student food service program that would offer "all you can eat 24 hours a day" for an additional $300 per semester above the regular dormitory food service fee? Probably only the defensive line of the football team. Such a plan would quickly go bankrupt, as have HMOs that have priced themselves in such a way as to attract only high-risk subscribers.

The financial incentives for both subscribers and physicians in an HMO encourage less costly outpatient alternatives to hospitalization. Outpatient expenses are fully covered for the HMO subscriber, whereas the individual with conventional hospital insurance coverage would have to pay such expenses out of pocket. Many HMOs also pay physicians bonuses from whatever surpluses exist as a result of lower utilization experience, thus providing a clear incentive for efficient patient management. In regular fee-for-service practice, the more services used, particularly costly hospital surgical services, the more money a physician makes.

**Gateway 2: Adjusting the Supply
of Health Manpower in an HMO**

Physician-to-population ratios in HMOs are markedly different from those in the general population. Not only do HMOs seem to get by with fewer physicians, the distribution of them is also significantly different. There are more general practitioners and internists in HMOs and fewer surgeons and superspecialists. HMOs also tend to select physicians whose practice patterns and habits contribute to the organization's efficiency goals. Hospitals are only beginning to pay attention to this factor. HMOs have generally been more willing to utilize nurse practitioners, physician assistants, and other allied health professionals in order to reduce their dependence on more costly physician manpower to do routine screening and preventive procedures.

Gateway 3: Adjusting Capital Expenditures in an HMO

Hospitals owned by HMOs appear to get by comfortably with bed-to-population ratios that are approximately half the national ratio. HMOs that do not own their own hospitals have become increasingly more reluctant to enter into affiliations and contracts with more costly teaching or newer facilities, in spite of the greater credibility and image of quality they convey. HMOs also appear to be more restrained than conventional hospitals in their investments in costly diagnostic and therapeutic equipment.

Gateway 4: Adjusting Research and Development in an HMO

In most of the larger HMOs there are research and development units that focus, predictably, on assessment of the cost effectiveness of various organizational arrangements for dealing with health problems.

These activities may involve relatively straightforward scheduling and staffing studies or more involved experimentation with new benefit packages or service programs. The Kaiser Foundation Health Plan, for example, has created an independent research unit; the unit has developed a large staff and data base and supplements its internal funding with outside research grants. Unlike most research in health settings, which focuses almost exclusively on clinical problems, the Kaiser group's efforts focus more on applied research in areas related to the efficient delivery of services.

Gateway 5: Adjusting the Production of Services in an HMO

The HMO is a vertically integrated system; that is, it offers services ranging from health promotion and illness prevention to treatment and rehabilitation. For this reason, it can alter both manpower mix and location of services to achieve the most cost-effective general treatment of illness for a population rather than concentrate on a particular, isolated episode that stimulated a visit or admission.

SUMMARY AND CONCLUSIONS:
FLEET FOOT'S FUTURE

Fleet Foot Hospital's future depends on its ability to manipulate effectively the five managerial control gateways. The real advantage that HMOs have in the present environment is the way they think about their control problems. They are used to operating in an environment with fixed resources, but there is no reason that hospitals cannot do the same. In order to reinforce this point, let us create an analogy.

Imagine that the health system is like the waterworks for a small town. The water in this case is money. Figure 2.4 provides a model of this system. There are two water towers that serve the town, one supplied by the general public. From this tower, water (funds) flows to a second tower, the third-party health insurance reserves, and to providers (out-of-pocket purchases of health services). The relative sizes of expenditures are represented by the relative sizes of providers' houses. Each house can continue to expand, adding extra bathrooms and so on, confident that there will always be enough water to flush the toilets. This works well until a drought ensues or until the community has expanded beyond the capacity of the water table to replenish the supply. The morning shower is reduced to a trickle. What is particularly disturbing to the people in the waterworks is that there is going to be an increasing number of people using these houses, and a lot of them will

Figure 2.4   Unrestricted Flow of Expenditures (1985 Estimates in Billions of Dollars)

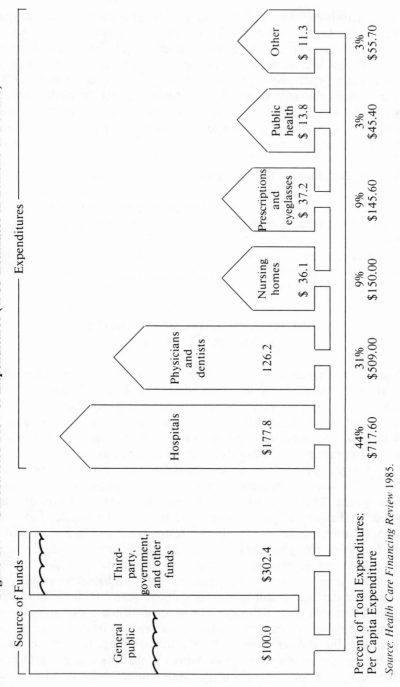

	Source of Funds		Expenditures					
	General public	Third-party, government, and other funds	Hospitals	Physicians and dentists	Nursing homes	Prescriptions and eyeglasses	Public health	Other
	$100.0	$302.4	$177.8	126.2	$36.1	$37.2	$13.8	$11.3

Percent of Total Expenditures: 44%   31%   9%   9%   3%   3%
Per Capita Expenditure $717.60 $509.00 $150.00 $145.60 $45.40 $55.70

Source: Health Care Financing Review 1985.

want to move into the nursing facilities. A water shortage is declared. Voluntary cooperation of the citizens is urged. No more watering the front lawn and only one shower a day. These measures are not sufficient, however, so a series of control valves is put in place (figure 2.5). Each can effectively restrict the supply of water, but each will have its own consequences for the members of the community.

The first control valve simply directs the flow of dollars from consumers, forcing them to ration expenditures for health services. To most people, the allocation of health services on the basis of ability to pay for them is morally repugnant, therefore other control valves are sought. The second control valve offers what seems to be a reasonable alternative. It involves creating a more competitive situation among health insurance carriers. Each would try to provide a fixed set of services at a fixed price for individuals and groups of employees. The third party would then play the role of rationer rather than consumer. Its effectiveness would determine its solvency and ability to attract subscribers. Providers, however, resist implementation of such controls—it seems to them to be a case of the tail wagging the dog. Consequently, a variety of other controls has been explored. For hospitals (the fourth control valve), this involves prospective reimbursement and, recently, flat-rate reimbursement on the basis of DRGs. Many of the controls focus on hospitals, since they represent the largest chunk of expenditures. Obviously, since no matter which of these valves is regulated there will not be enough "water" to supply all of these providers, some of them will be squeezed. Hospitals, physicians, nursing homes, and so on now compete directly with each other for scarce resources.

A variety of tactics has been used to assure hospitals' financial viability. Some of these windows of opportunity, however, have become windows of vulnerability. In the past, cost controls on hospitals were limited to controls on per diem costs. Many strategies are possible for hospitals in adjusting to these controls. First, length of stay per admission can be increased, spreading costs over a longer period and thus reducing average per diem costs. Perhaps partly as a result of this practice, the average length of stay, which had been dropping for 40 years, appeared stalled in many metropolitan areas; it dropped again dramatically only with the implementation of Medicare's DRG payment system. Utilization controls that disallowed some excessive stays and inappropriate admissions had been relatively ineffective in curbing this practice. In some state Medicaid programs where such disallowances have been applied extensively, they have generated more ill will than reduced length of stay. Another way of getting around controls on per diem costs is to alter the mix of patients away from cases with high per

Figure 2.5   Rationed Flow of Expenditures

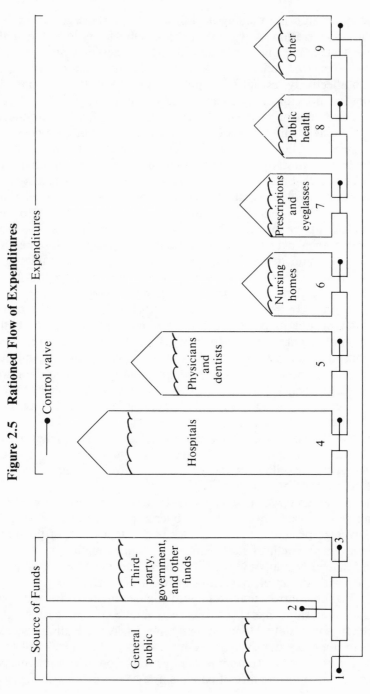

● Control valve

Source of Funds

Expenditures

General public

Third-party, government, and other funds

Hospitals   4

Physicians and dentists   5

Nursing homes   6

Prescriptions and eyeglasses   7

Public health   8

Other   9

Source: Health Care Financing Review 1985.

diem costs. This practice is more clearly visible among nursing homes, where facilities in some areas have competed aggressively for the "easy care" patients—that is, the patients who may not need to be in a nursing home in the first place.

Yet another alternative is to shift costs onto other payers. Privately insured or self-paying patients' charges can often be adjusted to take into account losses resulting from costs disallowed by third parties that pay on a cost basis. One of the problems with this approach is that it is not available to all hospitals. Inner-city hospitals and hospitals in poor rural areas are far more dependent on public cost-based third parties and have few bona fide private payers (those that actually pay charges instead of not paying at all). This discrepancy split the united front of hospitals in New Jersey and produced a system of uniform payments by all payers. The other problem with the approach is that it forces commercial carriers and self-paying patients to carry an inequitable share of the burden for a facility; in some states, particularly in the East, it has brought about the virtual abandonment of the health insurance market by commercial carriers. Pressures are mounting to alleviate both problems. The 1982 Medicare regulations impose ceilings on reimbursement based on diagnostic category, thus transforming extended lengths of stay for Medicare patients into a liability for the hospital rather than a windfall. Lobbyists for commercial insurance, often finding themselves allied with state hospital associations, have attempted to change state insurance laws and reduce or eliminate "contractual discounts" (the difference between allowed cost reimbursement and charges) given Blue Cross and public payers in their contracts with hospitals.

Assuming that these windows of opportunity are closed, Fleet Foot Hospital is going to have to engage in much fancier footwork. It will have to calculate returns and break-even points for the treatment of several diagnostic groups and alter its case mix accordingly. This can be done through selective recruitment of medical staff, more focused marketing, and "demarketing" (a new word in the hospital's vocabulary) of specific services. Demarketing involves restricting the volume of deficit-generating services, both by controlling portals of entry (elective admissions and emergency room services) and by restricting the number of beds and other physical resources available for the treatment of patients likely to generate bad debts.

This kind of fine tuning will probably fail to stem losses in the long run, since in both the New Jersey DRG program and the new Medicare regulations ceilings are based on peer group averages. These ceilings will presumbly drop, since all of the facilities will be attempting to achieve the same objective, and living under them will become increasingly onerous. Fleet Foot must move in two directions. First, it must find less expensive substitutes. Its situation is not unlike that of candy manufacturers a few years ago. Vending machines had a single, twenty-five cent slot for candy bars. Sugar prices doubled in a period of a year or so. The candy bar became a loss leader, since it could only be sold for twenty-five cents even though it actually cost substantially more. The solution? In the short run it was too costly to change the candy machines, so the candy bar itself was made smaller. In a hospital, that solution translates into more aides and licensed practical nurses on the floor instead of registered nurses, more ambulatory surgery centers, and so forth. Fleet Foot must shift its product line to a less costly one. If this is distasteful, the hospital has two other options. First, it can expand into uncontrolled markets. In general this means increasing its emphasis on outpatient services, possibly in direct competition with some of its medical staff. A second alternative is to develop new products and services—executive physicals, occupational health, meals on wheels—to offset whatever deficits it incurs in providing inpatient services. Some hospitals have spun off subsidiaries that have little or no connection to the provision of health care.

Ultimately, if Fleet Foot is going to survive with any degree of autonomy, it must become a regulator itself. There are a variety of ways this could be accomplished. It could set up its own HMO or enter into a risk-sharing arrangement with one. Fleet Foot would then make resource allocation decisions much like the restaurateur and the HMO developer described in the last section. Many capitation-based hospital reimbursement plans have been developed on an experimental, demonstration basis with local Blue Cross plans, and many hospitals have entered into these ventures independently.

On the other hand, Fleet Foot could decide that, rather than competing with the other providers for increasingly restricted financial resources, it would collaborate with them on the regional level. Hospitals in the Rochester area of New York State, for example, have entered into contracts with Blue Cross, Medicare, and Medicaid to develop a regional capitation program—in other words, a regional pot of money that the hospitals themselves allocate. Such a process presumably reverses incentives to maximize inpatient utilization and greatly encourages shared services within the region.

Clearly, Fleet Foot has some very important and difficult decisions to make. Whether it chooses the collaborative or the competitive course, it, along with other providers, will transform the existing health care system into something very different than what has existed before. In the next chapter, we review the outcomes of the current system that are making such basic changes inevitable.

3

Consequences

So oft in theologic wars,
    The disputants, I ween,
Rail on in utter ignorance
    Of what each other mean.
And prate about an Elephant
    Not one of them has seen.

John Godfrey Saxe (1979, 232)

In the last chapter we reviewed the gateways that the management component could use to control the allocation of resources. In this chapter we deal with what is perhaps an even more critical task of the management component, the assessment of performance.

As with the blind men and the elephant, much heated debate has surrounded the performance of the health system and its components. We first take stock of the trends in this performance and then look at some of the problems and the initiatives undertaken to solve them. Finally, we draw some conclusions about the potential effectiveness of these initiatives.

TRENDS IN PERFORMANCE OF THE HEALTH CARE LABYRINTH

I once asked a worker at a crematorium, who had a curiously contented look on his face, what he found so satisfying about his work. He replied that what fascinated him was the way in which so much went in and so little came out (Cochrane 1972, 12).

There are three distinct categories of output in a health system: (1) units of service, (2) dollars spent, and (3) health status. Assuming that society can reach some level of consensus on the measurement of each of these categories of output, there are five basic questions that can be raised in assessing the performance of the health system:

1. Are services *accessible*? (That is, are a sufficient number of units of service provided to meet the overall needs of the population?)

2. Are the costs incurred in the provision of those services *affordable*? (That is, are the total costs, given the other desires and needs of society, reasonable?)

3. Are these services provided *efficiently*? (That is, are the costs per unit of service or per person as low as possible?)

4. Are the services *effective*? (That is, do they produce the desired result in terms of improved health status?)

5. Is there *equity* in the distribution of such services and benefits? (That is, do different racial, income, geographic groups get a fair share of the benefits or costs of the existing system?)

These questions are all value laden. We can, however, come to some general conclusions, both objective and subjective, about the direction in which each of these aspects of performance is moving.

Accessibility

In the course of this century, individuals in the United States have received increasingly more health services. The average number of physician visits per year grew from about 2.6 per person in 1930 to 4.8 in 1980 (Donabedian, Axelrod, and Wyszewianski 1980, 35; National Center for Health Statistics 1983, 8). The site of these visits has shifted almost completely from the patient's home (about 40 percent of all visits in 1928) to physicians' offices and institutional settings. Use of acute-care hospitals has risen from 746 days per thousand persons in 1928 to about 1,290 days (Donabedian, Axelrod, and Wyszewianski 1980, 81). Hospital use has also shifted from a more custodial to a more production orientation. Between 1930 and the present, the number of discharges per thousand persons jumped from 59 to 167, and the average length of stay dropped from 12.7 days to 6.9 (Donabedian, Axelrod, and Wyszewianski 1980, 81; National Center for Health Statistics 1984, 3). At the same time, the number and type of both providers of individual services and institutional services have expanded.

Subjective perceptions have generally identified the same shifts. Concerns about a physician shortage and access to adequate hospital care in rural areas in the early 1960s have been supplanted with concerns about physician oversupply and "overbeddedness" in the 1980s [excess national bed capacity has been estimated at over 100,000 (Vignola 1979)]. Physician supply, which has risen rapidly in the last 15 years, is projected to increase further, to an unprecedented 259.6 active physicians per 100,000 population by the year 2000 (U.S. Department of Health and Human Services 1985b). The lack of responsiveness of providers to community needs also appears to be far less heated an issue than it used to be. Medical schools have placed greater emphasis on training primary care physicians, and at least some of the energies of acute-care hospitals have shifted toward preventive, community programs. Their recent concern with marketing has perhaps done as much to make hospitals responsive to community needs as three generations of regional planning agencies did.

There are still, however, serious problems in terms of access. For example, a study by The Robert Wood Johnson Foundation (Myers 1983) estimated that in 1982 some 300,000 U.S. families had a member who was refused medical care. While various diagnostic and surgical procedures are readily available to most people in this country, adequate care for the chronically ill, particularly for the poor, is in short supply. Further, the kind of caring rather than curing needed for the terminally ill and incurable is sorely lacking, as suggested by the following commentary by Daniel S. Barash, a victim of amyotrophic lateral sclerosis (ALS), a fatal degenerative syndrome marked by muscular weakness, atrophy, and spasticity:

I made an appointment with Dr. A. when next available, a month later. In the meantime I silently worried. I found a brief description of ALS as ". . . relentless and cruel," and told myself it wasn't that bad if I wouldn't let it be that bad. What I truly needed most was reassurance from Dr. A. I arrived that day to consult with Dr. A. about routine matters first, including my high blood pressure. Then, in his style, he counterfeited a question: What did I intend to do now that amyotrophic lateral sclerosis was diagnosed? I was set back, bewildered. What did he mean by "What am I going to do?" Some people travel and enjoy themselves, he said. Yes? What was he getting to? He then informed me, starkly, closing the door that his colleague, Dr. B., had left ambiguously ajar for a month, that my life expectancy with amyotrophic lateral sclerosis was two to four years. Silence. And that was it, after some more surface conversation, as far as Dr. A. and all of the HMO was concerned. Our responsibility is at an end, nice knowing you, go home and kick off (Barash 1984, 13).

Affordability

The most dramatic changes in health care costs have taken place in the acute-care hospital: just since 1965, costs per stay have increased more than eightfold. The percentage of the GNP going for health care tells a similar story: since 1929, it has risen from 3.5 to 10.6 percent in 1984. Annual per capita expenditures for health care, adjusted for inflation, have grown from less than $50 to over $1,580 in the same period (U.S. Department of Health and Human Services 1985a).

Affordability, of course, is relative to what one has to spend. As the GNP rises, the percentage spent on health services, as on other "luxury" items, rises (Getzen 1981). Indeed, the very close relationship between GNP and expenditures for health care raises the question of whether these expenditures are really out of control at all. What has made the question of affordability a public issue rather than simply one of consumer preference is the increase in the public share of these expenditures on health care. Public funds accounted for more than 40 percent of all expenditures in the post-Medicare and Medicaid years. The implications of allowing such drastic increases in health costs to continue during a period of slow economic growth and burgeoning public debt are perceived by most policymakers as politically and economically unthinkable. As a result, 1983 saw a major shift toward fixed reimbursements for providers under the Medicare program. Restrictions on costs are likely to become tighter as competition for scarce public dollars increases.

The overall increase in the proportion of the population with some third-party insurance coverage, as well as the increasing portion of the bill being covered by third parties, has softened the impact of these cost increases on the individual consumer. All third parties combined (private health insurers, government, and industry) now finance 72 percent of all personal health care; they cover 91 percent of hospital care, 72 percent of physicians' services, and 44 percent of the remaining health services (U.S. Department of Health and Human Services 1985a). Yet for some individuals, affordability remains a problem. As a result of cutbacks in benefits, individual consumers are becoming responsible for a greater proportion of expenditures. Even more serious, 21 to 27 million persons remain uncovered by third-party programs (Stevens 1983, 32).

Efficiency

Faced with a cost-income squeeze, productivity has become a paramount concern. The signs here are not particularly encouraging, however.

In terms of hospital productivity, there has been a steady increase in the number of full-time-equivalent staff per patient-day since 1965. Some observers argue that these increases have been compensated for, in part, by faster throughput, which has resulted in a progressive decline in average length of stay. Reduction in length of stay, however, is not a particularly useful indicator of enhanced system efficiency. There are striking differences in average length of stay between California and New York, yet expenditures on Medicare enrollees, adjusted for age and sex differences, are almost identical. (The shorter average length of stay in California is mitigated by higher per diem costs and higher expenditures on outpatient care rendered by physicians.)

Evidence of increased productivity in physicians' office practices is not much more encouraging. In general, estimates of increased productivity have ranged from 1 percent to 3 percent per year (National Center for Health Statistics 1979, 3). These increases reflect the gradual elimination of the house call and a gradual increase in the number of nonphysician staff hired in physicians' offices. Evidence does not suggest that increases in the number of physicians working in group practices and HMOs are likely to lead to increases in productivity. Most of the conventional measures and thinking about productivity are somewhat inappropriate when applied to physicians, who are largely self-employed. A "backward-bending supply of hours" appears to describe physician behavior: physicians seem to be willing to expand the number of hours they work until they reach their desired income level, after which they taper off. Also, most of the costs of an office visit are physician-generated; therefore, as the market begins to be saturated with physicians and the number of patients per physician declines, services for those patients tend to become more elaborate, and output per physician tends to be lower and more costly.

The public generally perceives the health system as inefficient. Legislators, policymakers, and corporate leaders want to encourage efficiency, and their concern is reflected in the implementation of such efficiency-inducing approaches to reimbursement in public programs as Medicare and Medicaid. Corporations, concerned about the escalating costs of health care benefits for their employees and the impact those expenditures have on their expenses, have formed coalitions to explore ways of controlling costs. Among the options are self-insured capitation, preferred provider relationships, and increased deductibles and coinsurance for employees. Even labor unions, which championed the creation of extended health insurance benefits in this country, have, in some areas, joined these efforts. Pressures from the public, corporations, and unions, based on their perception that the health care system is inefficient, are a driving force for change.

Effectiveness

> Quality is the last refuge of the physician
> when all other arguments fail.
>
> Ernest Saward (1976)

If the costs of services are increasing and the efficiency with which they are provided is, or may be, declining, what are we getting in return? Since so much hinges on the answer to this question, we will explore in some detail the assessment of effectiveness. In the past, effectiveness, or quality of care (we will assume, for the purposes of this discussion, that the two terms are identical), has been an accelerator, forcing rapid cost increases in the health system. It seems likely that it will now serve as a brake, slowing structural changes that might enhance efficiency or affordability. Can something as subjective and ephemeral as effectiveness or quality be measured at all? Clinicians, managers, third-party insurers, and legislators are expected to protect the public by doing just that. The process they have devised to measure quality involves reviews that become progressively more rigorous, costly, and time-consuming to carry out. This review, or search, process is summarized in figure 3.1.

The simplest way of assuring quality or effectiveness is simply to look at *structure*, or inputs. One must determine whether resources assumed to be associated with effectiveness are present and whether they are organized in a way that is also assumed to be associated with effectiveness. For example, one can look at the credentials of the staff, the fire resistance of the building, and the bylaws and committee structure of the medical staff and come to some conclusions about whether more effective care is likely to take place in such an environment. This is essentially the approach of such outside certifying bodies as state licensure boards and the Joint Commission on Accreditation of Hospitals. Neither of these bodies, of course, provides any guarantee that effective care takes place, only that, in its professional judgment, effective care is more likely or less likely to take place.

An assessment of structure may be sufficient for some forms of external evaluation, but it is clearly insufficient for assessing the internal

Figure 3.1 Search Procedures for Determining Health Care Effectiveness

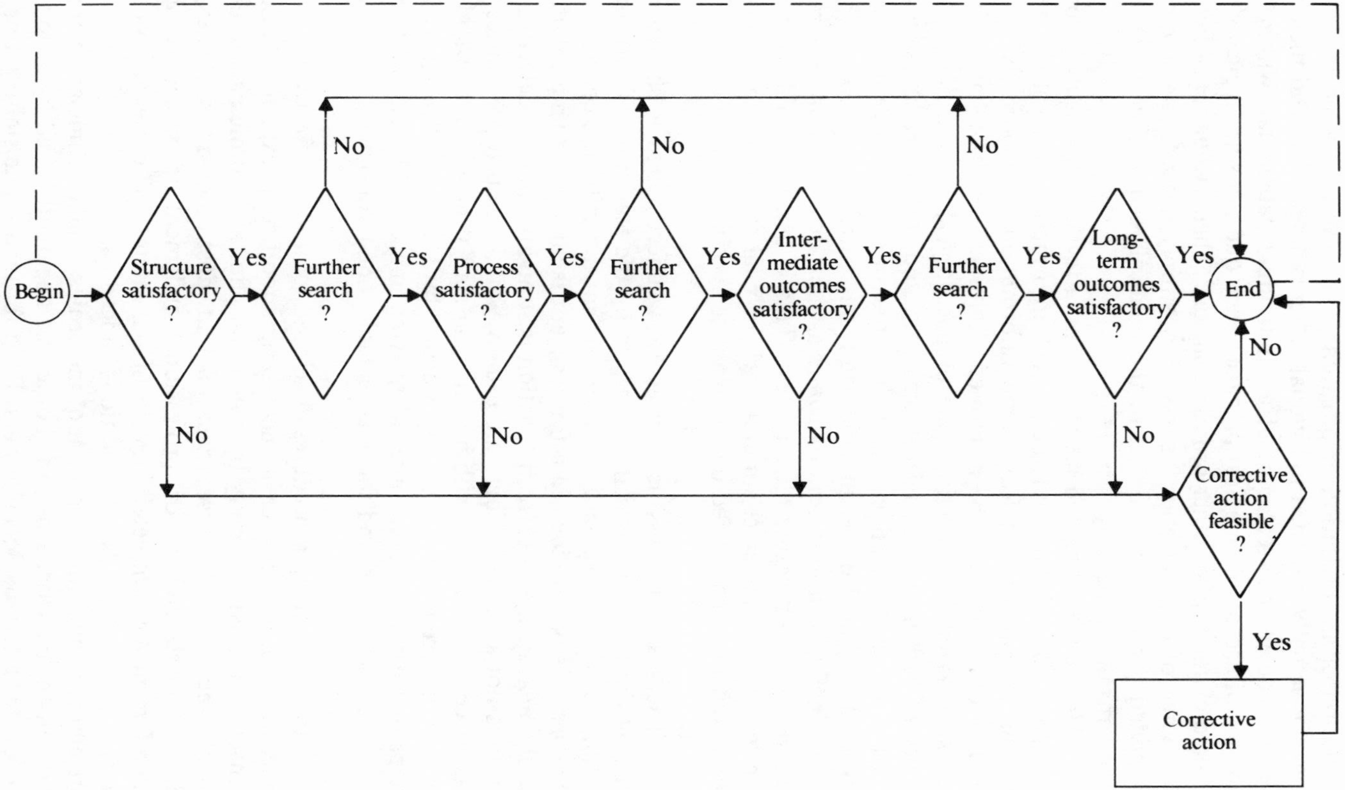

operation of an institution or program. There must be some review of the care actually provided individual patients, or *process*. Did the decisions made in the treatment of an individual patient fall within the bounds of acceptable medical practice? Such questions are typically answered by medical or other professional staff. Their evaluations offer no guarantee of optimal effectiveness, they simply indicate that the care provided (or at least recorded in the medical record) met acceptable standards of practice.

Most institutions and programs, and a few outside certifying bodies, have moved beyond relying on such informal and subjective mechanisms to collecting at least some information on *intermediate outcomes*, or what have been termed "sentinel health events." Such statistics as rate of infection, rate of postsurgical complications, incidence of bedsores, incidence of accidents, and rate of readmission are used to measure effectiveness. If these measures rise above acceptable levels, they should trigger in-depth study and corrective action.

Finally, such *long-term outcomes* as mortality and morbidity rates can be used to measure effectiveness. This is usually feasible only on the level of the larger community, where vital statistics can be monitored and research carried out to evaluate specific treatments and programs.

The search process used in assessing effectiveness is shaped not just by the resources available, but also by the feasibility of corrective action. It is relatively easy, for example, for a certifying body to insist that services be provided in a fire-resistant facility. Such an attribute is easily measured, and corrective action is straightforward: a defective facility is not approved. There are usually well-developed procedures for taking corrective action within a medical staff if process reviews identify an unacceptable pattern of practice by someone. The corrective steps that would be taken after identifying unacceptable sentinel health events are less clear, and for unacceptable long-term outcomes they are still less clear.

In the practical procedures developed to monitor effectiveness, the rules of scientific evidence are necessarily modified by expediency. Consensus is arrived at simply by relying on clinical or professional judgment. There are, of course, trade-offs that must be made for this expediency. First, clinical or professional judgment is subjective and therefore never completely devoid of self-interest. There is always the danger that standards or conditions judged essential for effectiveness are actually more for the benefit of the professional or clinician than the patient. In one case, a nursing home was apparently cited by state surveyors for a serious deficiency and fined for inadequate staffing, not because there was inadequate staffing in terms of patient care, but because a registered nurse was expected to clean bathtubs on the weekend shift. Another home was judged deficient because there was no window in the social worker's office (Smith 1981). Second, since the standards rely on subjective judgment and are tied only tenuously to outcome, they have often proved exceedingly difficult to enforce within the legal system. Both of these trade-offs surface again in our discussion of organizational structures.

Improvements in effectiveness, in professionally defined standards, or structure, have nevertheless been exceptional. As described briefly in chapter 1, the credentialing and staffing requirements of institutional providers have shifted strikingly, as have requirements regarding medical staff control over practice within institutional settings. The physical structure and organization of hospitals have changed significantly since the passage of Medicare and Medicaid. These bills imposed many requirements and standards on hospitals in the areas of records, staffing, and physical construction. The changes in long-term care facilities are even more dramatic, since they have taken place in a far shorter period of time.

Some indicators also suggest positive effects on long-term outcomes. Life expectancy has increased progressively in this century, leveling off somewhat in the 1950s but accelerating again in the 1970s. Between 1957 and 1967 one year was added to the expected lifespan of a child born in the United States, while between 1967 and 1977 two years were added (Rice 1978).

Although the rate of neonatal mortality declined only 12 percent from 1950 to 1965, it declined 35 percent in the next decade. Between 1950 and 1965, the annual rate of decline in neonatal mortality was lower for nonwhites than for whites, but it shifted to 50 percent higher for nonwhites during the subsequent ten years (Lee et al. 1980, 16). These drops are not explained by any significant shifts in birth weight, the most significant predictor of neonatal mortality. Improved perinatal care since 1965, particularly for women in low-income groups, appears to be the most plausible explanation.

An analysis comparing per capita health care expenditures to mortality rates in some 400 county groupings in the United States in 1970 came to similar conclusions concerning the efficacy of increases in health care expenditures. A 10 percent increase in medical care expenditures was associated with an average 1.57 percent decrease in mortality rates (Hadley 1982, 8).

In general, there is limited evidence that changes in health care affect long-term outcomes. Even the introduction of antibiotics in the

1940s, popularly assumed to have greatly reduced the number of deaths from infectious diseases, appears not to have accelerated the decline in mortality for most such diseases (Hemminkis and Paakkulainen 1976). A study in Los Angeles County in January 1976 actually concluded that the reduction in surgical procedures and the restriction of other services produced by a malpractice insurance crisis probably produced a net reduction in the mortality rate (James 1979).

More damaging is the fact that often, even when there is evidence that reallocating resources would increase the likelihood of desirable long-term outcomes, such changes have not been made. For example, even in the face of strong clinical evidence that mental patients can be treated effectively without being institutionalized, admission rates of psychiatric hospitals have increased over the last two years and the bias toward inappropriate institutional treatment appears to remain (Kiewsler 1982). Similarly, although widely accepted policy studies have advocated greater emphasis on preventive and environmental programs instead of curative ones, there has generally been no shift toward them (Evans 1982). Another example: after years of heated debate, legislation mandating airbags in new cars has never been passed, even though the death rate from traffic accidents continues to be appallingly high. Efforts to reduce morbidity and mortality resulting from occupational hazards have improved conditions somewhat, but byssinosis, asbestosis, and other diseases continue to take their toll—even though preventing them would cost society less in the long run.

The momentum toward greater effectiveness now seems to be slowing. Quality of care appears to be receding further and further from the consciousness of administrators, third parties, legislative bodies, and administrative agencies. Deregulation is a more pressing concern than quality assurance. Proposed regulations for Medicare certification recently suggested that nursing homes receive the same option to use JCAH accreditation for participation in Medicare as acute-care hospitals and that a more flexible schedule of inspection be created for them. In the storm of protest that ensued, a legislative freeze was imposed, pending further study. The financial incentives of fixed charges, as opposed to cost-based reimbursement, will no doubt slow the movement toward quality assurance even more, as will the lack of clear connections between standards and outcomes.

More recent indicators of long-term outcome portend reductions in effectiveness. Infant mortality has increased in several urban areas. Moreover, several urban areas document a rising percentage of women who have received little or no prenatal care. The 4.6 percent per year average rate of decline in infant mortality between 1965 and 1982 slowed to less than 2 percent in 1983 and 1984, and many observers believe the change is related to cuts in funding for maternal and child health programs (Pear 1985, 1). These reductions, coupled with reductions in Aid to Families with Dependent Children and Medicaid eligibility among 200,000 working mothers because of changes in eligibility requirements, fewer food stamps for 1 million persons, and reduced benefits for 250,000 women and children in federal nutrition programs, suggest the potential for even greater increases in infant mortality (Myers 1983).

Equity

How have these shifts in overall access, expenditure, and effectiveness affected equity? Have the gaps between various ethnic and income groups closed or widened?

Dramatic, perhaps even revolutionary, changes have taken place in equity of access since the passage of Medicare and Medicaid in 1965. For example, the number of physician visits per person per year for the lowest income group increased from 3.9 to 5.9 between 1964 and 1983, whereas the opposite effect obtained in the highest income group (U.S. Department of Health and Human Services 1984, 82).

Similar shifts have taken place in hospital usage. Between 1956 and 1974, the number of days spent in hospital per thousand persons per year significantly increased for all income groups without private hospital insurance, except for persons in the highest income category. As one would expect, the most striking increase in utilization has taken place in the lowest income group, among persons without private health insurance. Here the rate of hospital use has doubled since 1965, from 1,000 days in hospital per thousand persons per year to 2,000. However, the number of people among the low-income group unable to pay for hospital care because of inadequate funds or lack of insurance is growing steadily. Between 1979 and 1982, a 20.9 percent increase in this group was noted. During this time provision of free care by hospitals increased by only 3.8 percent (Feder and Hadley 1984, 545), and there has been an upsurge in hospitals' dumping of patients who cannot pay for services (*Wall Street Journal* 1985, 33). Also, the percent of black mothers obtaining early prenatal care dropped between 1980 and 1983 (Ingram et al. 1986). The gap between whites and blacks, which had narrowed in the previous decade, began to widen.

Whether these shifts have closed the gap in equity of access or not is difficult to assess. Income and health status are highly correlated, but the relative differences in number of visits to a physician per person per year are only a blurred reflection of this correlation. The patterns of utilization remain strikingly different between low- and high-income groups. A disproportionate share of low-income persons' visits to physicians are to outpatient clinics, where services tend to be episodic or disease-oriented and continuity or coordination is limited. The poor who see a private physician are likely to travel 20 percent farther and wait 40 percent longer (Davis, Gold, and Makuc 1981, 169). The most striking differences in utilization patterns by income are in dental and preventive services, which have been least affected by recent public reimbursement schemes. Frequency of visits to a dentist remains directly related to income. Fewer persons in the lowest income groups see a physician for routine physicals, and twice the number of low-income respondents reported an interval of more than two years since their last visit (U.S. Department of Health and Human Services 1984, 86). Black women (with proportionally lower income than white women) generally see a physician later in their pregnancy, have fewer prenatal care visits, and experience two to three times the risk of negative birth outcomes, low birth weight, and higher infant death and morbidity rates than white women (Institute of Medicine 1985, 51). Black women are also less likely than white women to receive diagnostic X rays (10.8 pecent versus 13.5 percent) and ultrasound procedures (4.5 percent versus 4.9 percent) during pregnancy (U.S. Department of Health and Human Services 1984, 35). Poor women are 40 percent less likely to have had the benefit of a breast examination for early detection of cancer than women from higher income groups (Davis, Gold, and Makuc 1981, 170).

Expenditures for health care by income and racial group also reflect the shifts brought about by increased public financing of health services. Overall out-of-pocket expenditures continue to be higher in upper-income groups, even though the proportion of family income spent on health services is lower. Public financing, however, now absorbs these discrepancies, producing mean total expenditures that are highest in the lowest income category.

Nevertheless, some differences in equity of expenditures remain. Study of Medicare beneficiaries is useful for determining differences in expenditure by income and race, because all beneficiaries have identical comprehensive benefits. Expenditures of nonwhites for physician and outpatient services are about 30 percent lower per enrollee than expenditures of whites; they are 20 percent lower per enrollee for inpatient services (National Center for Health Statistics 1979). Medicare recipients in the lowest income category, although more likely to need aid, received less than half the dollar amount in benefits under the supplementary medical insurance program (part B) that those in the highest income category received (U.S. Department of Health, Education, and Welfare 1978, 271). These differences appear to result from structural factors rather than discriminatory policies of insurance plans or individual providers: the medical care infrastructure is more limited and more poorly developed in areas with a low-income, nonwhite population. Areas with lower per capita income and education have, predictably, significantly fewer physicians, hospital beds, and other resources per thousand persons.

The gap in life expectancy between whites and nonwhites has narrowed in this century. A nonwhite could expect to live only 65 percent as long as a white at the turn of the century; he or she now enjoys a life expectancy that is 93 percent of that of a white person. This shift probably reflects the marked declines in infant and neonatal death rates.

The issue of equity is now focused on cost shifting and differential rates of reimbursement embedded in current third-party reimbursement practices rather than on equity in access to health services. The time-honored Robin Hood principle, which has helped assure greater equity of access, is being challenged. Private paying patients and those with commercial coverage have traditionally paid substantially higher rates for services than Medicare and Medicaid patients, thus providing a hidden subsidy. Legislation is being proposed and enacted at the state level to prohibit this practice.

REASSESSING OVERALL PERFORMANCE

In order to assess overall performance of a system, one must come up with a way of weighting and combining assessments of accessibility, affordability, efficiency, effectiveness, and equity. The weights given these attributes will change as society redefines what health care is. As we suggested in chapter 1, such definitions go through cycles of change as the adverse consequences of a particular definition become clearer. We have recently gone through a period where health care has been defined predominantly as a professional service, an effort to synthesize the notions of health care as an economic good and as a social relationship. As a consequence, we have achieved in the last 50 years dramatic improvements in access, equity, and, to a lesser extent, effectiveness. We have paid for these improvements with serious reductions in both affordability and efficiency. As a result, health care now appears to be defined as more of an economic good, and efforts are being made to restructure the health care system in order to improve efficiency and affordability. The critical questions now are, how high a price for this latest shift are we going to have to pay, and in the long run will we be willing to pay it?

PROGNOSIS

The patient (the U.S. health care system) is now undergoing treatment. Part of the treatment is a major restructuring of the system into a larger, more centralized, corporate form, as described in chapter 1. The other part of the treatment is a change in the manner of payment, from fee-for-service to capitation, as described in chapter 2. These are the most commonly advocated treatments for the lack of efficiency and affordability in the system. Will they succeed in eliminating or at least alleviating the problems without causing serious side effects? Are we, like nineteenth century physicians, providing a cure that is no more advanced than bleeding or purging? Like any good practitioner, we must review the evidence carefully before recommending a treatment. We devote the remainder of this chapter to a review of what capitation payment and corporate structure may contribute to improving the efficiency and affordability of health care.

Corporately Structured Multi-institutional Systems

In chapter 1 we mentioned four shifts that have taken place in the organization of health care: (1) increased size of provider units, (2) increased specialization of services, (3) increased centralization of control through the development of multi-institutional systems, and (4) greater private ownership. Are these shifts part of the solution to the performance problems of the health system, as has been claimed, or are they simply part of the problem?

Underlying most of the arguments for the enhanced efficiency produced by these structural shifts is the assumption that the health sector is still a relatively undeveloped cottage industry that could become substantially more efficient if its structure were similar to that of the industrial sector. The central assumption is that substantial gains in efficiency can be obtained by operating on a larger scale. In general, economies of scale result from (1) the law of large numbers, which assures more stable demand, less random fluctuation, and consequently less idle capacity; (2) economies of bulk transactions, such as sales and purchasing; and (3) the indivisibility of inputs that come in whole units and are less costly per use if used to capacity (Hefty 1969). These assumed economies of scale could be achieved through growth of individual institutions, more specialization of services, or merger.

Economies of scale are more problematic in health-related institutions than in industry. First, many health care providers experience relatively little random fluctuation in demand. Nursing homes, for example, usually operate at almost peak capacity. Occupancy rates for smaller nursing homes are actually higher than occupancy rates for hospitals, which face more complex, segmented demand (Sirrocco 1981, 3). Even in large hospitals that have high occupancy rates, other factors generally produce substantially higher costs per unit of service. There also appears to be very little opportunity for economies of scale in physician group practices, and then only in practices with fewer than five physicians.

The potential economies of bulk transactions also appear less relevant. Certificate-of-need controls on supply generally make the recruitment of patients relatively simple and give no special advantage to larger operations. The preference of patients for services close to home may give smaller, more widely diffused facilities a competitive advantage. Also, the predominance of third parties such as Medicaid in the financing of services provides for uniform bulk financial transactions with providers, regardless of their size. Economies of bulk purchasing of supplies and personnel, to the extent that they exist, do not require large institutions, only shared-service and group-purchasing arrangements. There are nevertheless certain inputs, such as specialized staff, that are indivisible and require a certain number of patients in order to be used to full capacity. Accreditation, licensure, and certification procedures for Medicare and Medicaid reimbursement largely determine the cost-effective size of facilities. Smaller facilities cannot justify the employment of specialized staff on a full-time basis and have to contract such services out, which may make the services more costly. Advanced technology, which requires a high volume of utilization in order to be cost-effective, also affects size.

There are a number of reasons why one should not expect economies of scale in the provision of health services. First, the cost of travel restricts the size of facilities that will be used to capacity. Close to 70 percent of consumers select the physician and the hospital that are geographically closest to them (Weiss and Greenlick 1970). Even in metropolitan areas hospital choice is strongly influenced by distance (McGuirk and Porelli 1984). Similar preferences, to the extent that choice is available, seem likely to influence occupancy of other kinds of facilities. Second, as facilities and systems become larger, they become more vulnerable to the inefficiencies imposed upon them by their professional staffs (Roemer and Shonick 1973). Growth is perceived as an opportunity to acquire more costly, specialized services rather than to increase efficiency. The complex, specialized teaching center is the model to which professional staffs aspire. Many diseconomies of scale may be caused by professional and, consequently, regulatory pressures on smaller facilities to mimic the cost and complexity of larger ones. Finally, given the geographic restrictions on utilization of services, growth enhances monopolistic control over the provision of services and therefore produces a lack of concern for efficiency.

Empirical studies have generally concluded that economies of scale in the health sector are either nonexistent or insignificant. In nursing homes, costs per resident-day are directly related to the size of the facility: the larger the facility, the higher the costs (Sirrocco 1981, 16). Efforts to analyze economies of scale have attempted to control for some of the regional cost and product differences that mask the underlying relationship between size and costs. An analysis of the cost data from three states for different years and of a national survey that excluded capital-related expenses found that costs fell until a facility reached about 40 beds and that no additional economies were achievable in larger facilities (Birnbaum et al. 1981). A detailed study of operating costs in New York State concluded that economies of scale were generally of minimal importance and were essentially nonexistent in facilities with more than 50 beds (Lee and Birnbaum 1983).

The increase in size of acute-care hospitals and nursing homes has been closely associated with increases in cost. How much of these cost increases was related to increases in size rather than to advancements in technology would be difficult to determine. The strong association between them, however, raises the suspicion that some diseconomies of scale may be hidden in the cross-sectional analyses that have attempted to estimate the effects of changes in scale on efficiency.

Significant relationships have been found between ownership and cost for nursing homes. Costs per day for proprietary facilities, after attempting to adjust for other characteristics of these facilities, tend to be significantly lower than costs for voluntary or public facilities (Meiners 1982, Birnbaum et al. 1981, Lee and Birnbaum 1983).

In contrast, proprietary hospital facilities have been reported to have significantly higher costs and charges than voluntary hospitals (Lewin, Derzon, and Margulies 1981). Similar results were obtained in a comparison of investor-owned and voluntary facilities in California (Pattison and Katz 1983). Public hospitals in California that were managed under contract by investor-owned firms experienced significant increases in expenses per patient-day (Rundall and Lambert 1984).

Centralization does not appear to produce consistently greater efficiencies. In nursing homes, for example, centralization was found to be insignificantly but positively associated with costs (Meiners 1982). Similarly, acute-care hospital systems have little, if any, mitigating effect on overall costs for local communities (Zuckerman 1979). An evaluation of 16 shared-service organizations found that several of them actually increased members' costs (Health Services Research Center 1977). A study of hospital mergers concluded that, at least in urban areas, they tend to produce diseconomies (Treat 1976). Corporate (investor-owned) hospital systems have been found to exhibit higher total charges per adjusted patient-day than freestanding voluntary hospitals (Watt et al. 1986). A study by the General Accounting Office identified dramatic increases in capital costs (that is, in those reimbursed by Medicare) when facility ownership was transferred to multi-institutional systems (General Accounting Office 1983). According to advocates of multi-institutional systems, those systems that integrate services vertically (providing acute, rehabilitative, long-term, and primary care) rather than horizontally (providing similar services dispersed throughout a wide geographic area) offer a far greater opportunity for cost savings. Yet the preponderance of mergers and multi-institutional systems involve horizontal integration only. One review concludes that multi-institutional hospital systems increase the cost of care and that this increase is greater in for-profit than in not-for-profit systems (Ermann and Gabel 1984).

While increased specialization is often assumed to be associated with improved efficiency, it has been almost uniformly associated with higher costs in the health sector. Incomes of subspecialists, for example, are one-and-a-half times those of generalists (Owens 1979). Per diem costs in highly specialized teaching hospitals are two to three times those in typical general community hospitals. In a study of surgical admissions to 17 hospitals, in which results were adjusted for case mix, it was found that more specialized hospitals provided more intensive services for a longer time but with no appreciable difference in outcome (Scott, Hood, and Ewy 1979). Most studies of surgical performance have found a significant positive relationship between the number of procedures performed in a facility and positive outcomes. Such conclusions have been used by certificate-of-need and licensing agencies to establish volume criteria for specialized surgical programs in hospitals. One study, using discharge abstracts from 1,200 hospitals, found that, once the volume of procedures is controlled, hospital size is *negatively* related to outcome (Flood, Scott, and Ewy 1984).

In general, there appears to be little convincing evidence that the structural shifts in health care toward private ownership, greater centralization, and greater specialization have anything to do with achieving greater economies; nor do capitation arrangements assure greater system efficiency. We may indeed be offering treatments that are no more advanced than bleeding and purging.

Capitation Payment

Health maintenance organizations in various forms have long been advocated as a more effective means of delivering care. In general, researchers have found that most of the lower costs of HMOs result from the lower hospitalization rates of their members. Members of HMOs do not use significantly more outpatient services than other insured groups, nor are their costs per visit any less (Luft 1981). Researchers have generally found little in the way of economies of scale in physician practice, and comparisons of HMO and non-HMO outpatient expenses tend to confirm this.

The question is, how do HMOs reduce the hospitalization rates of their members? There are two ways: (1) selective enrollment of low-risk populations and (2) financial incentives for both enrollees and physicians to utilize services on an outpatient basis. From the perspective of the HMO, it does not really matter how the reduced hospitalization is achieved; indeed, other things being equal, the selective enrollment approach is more desirable, since it is less disruptive of patients' and physicians' existing habits and routines of care. From the point of view of the system as a whole, of course, it makes a good deal of difference. The critical question is whether the efficiencies (reduced rates of hospitalization) are real, or just another example of cost shifting and cream skimming.

There have been surprisingly few controlled comparisons of the hospitalization rates of subscribers before and after having the opportunity to join an HMO. Simply making age- and sex-adjusted comparisons of hospitalization rates between HMO and non-HMO subscribers is not unlike the blind men arguing about the elephant. Nine studies have included estimates of risk selection, based either on comparisons of pre-enrollment hospitalization rates (days in hospital per 1,000 persons) or measures of the health status of persons joining and persons not joining HMOs. Some HMOs were able to lower hospitalization rates significantly, whereas others were not. In most, risk selection played a greater role than internal efficiencies in determining the HMO's hospitalization experience. We summarize the nine studies briefly.

West Coast Medicare. This study by Eggers (1980) of a large West Coast prepaid group practice reported strikingly lower risk selection into the prepaid plan and has raised serious questions about the advisability of Medicare's entering into capitation arrangements with HMOs. The hospitalization rate for Medicare beneficiaries before selecting the HMO was only 38 percent of that for those not selecting the HMO. It appears that, in an elderly population where many very high risk individuals have preexisting ties to a practice and where outpatient care is already covered under Medicare, capitation is less likely to bring about internal efficiencies.

Washington, D.C., Medicaid. While lower risk selection into the prepaid group practice appears to have taken place, alteration of reimbursement incentives appears to have produced more internal efficiencies in terms of hospitalization (Gaus and Fuller 1972). The hospitalization rate of persons selecting the HMO was 55 percent of the rate of the control group, and over half that advantage appears attributable to internal efficiencies.

National Medicaid. This assessment of a variety of Medicaid capitation arrangements (Gaus, Cooper, and Hirschman 1976) generally supports the conclusions of the Washington, D.C., study and illustrates the possible differential effects of independent practice associations (IPAs) as opposed to prepaid groups. The health status measures may not accurately assess risk selection in terms of hospitalization; the ability of IPA enrollees to keep the physician they had prior to enrollment helps explain why IPAs are less effective in lowering hospitalization rates. Part of their ability to achieve lower hospitalization rates than the control populations, however, would seem attributable to the Medicaid program's reimbursement system, which encourages hospitalization.

Mountain Bell Blue Cross. Substantial internal efficiencies and less difference in risk selection appear to have been achieved by this large, prepaid group practice (Mitchell and Dunn 1978). Neither prior physician ties nor financial incentives appear sufficient in themselves to explain these results, which seem to be more clearly attributable to other internal efficiencies.

Rochester Blue Cross. Prior physician ties appear to be a significant factor in explaining the differential risk selection into the three plans offered (Sorensen et al. 1979). The IPA established through the local medical society enabled individuals to take advantage of the prepayment capitation arrangement without changing physician. Since physicians continued to be paid on a fee-for-service basis for the small proportion of their practices enrolled in the IPA, there was no financial incentive to restrict hospitalization. On the other hand, physicians in the prepaid group, whose incomes were dependent on the long-term financial viability of the plan, were able to work out ways of achieving internal efficiencies in terms of hospitalization. Thus, while the prepaid group was able to achieve an overall hospitalization rate of 51 percent of the control Blue Cross population, the IPA hospitalization rate was 236 percent of the control.

Selected California Standard Metropolitan Statistical Areas. This study attempted to measure the long-term impact of mature HMOs in a region where there is relatively large enrollment in some of the older plans (Blumberg 1980). Data from the National Health Interview Survey are used to compare health status and, consequently, likelihood of hospitalization for HMO and nonHMO enrollees. While lower hospitalization rates existed in the HMO population, survey data suggested that this group had a slightly higher risk of illness. This effect, one could argue, is caused by the settling effect in older HMOs. The initial impact of prior physician relationships washes out over time, and economic vulnerability plays a more important role in the differences in risk between prepaid and private insurance populations and the eventual effectiveness of reimbursement incentives in achieving internal efficiencies. The hospitalization rates of those in HMOs was only 78 percent of those enrolled in conventional private insurance plans.

Marshfield Clinic. In this particular study (Broida et al. 1975), financial incentives were the same for all physicians, since they were all salaried members of the clinic. There was a strong financial incentive for persons at risk of illness to join the prepaid plan, since it would not require any change of provider and, once enrolled, members could take advantage of its benefits. Thus, the prepaid group had hospitalization rates of 147 percent of the fee-for-service population.

Minneapolis–St. Paul Blue Cross–Blue Shield. An analysis of 11 Minneapolis–St. Paul employee groups during the year before optional HMO enrollment became available indicated that persons who subsequently enrolled in an HMO spent roughly half as much time in the hospital as those who retained fee-for-service coverage (470 days per 1,000 persons as opposed to 994) (Jackson-Beeck and Kleinman 1983). Expenditures on both hospitals and physicians were lower among those who subsequently selected HMO enrollment. The differences remained for all age groups, suggesting that self-selection was an important determinant of the differences in use and costs between persons with HMO coverage and persons with fee-for-service coverage.

Rand–Group Health Cooperative. A controlled trial in an established prepaid group practice was conducted to isolate the relation between prepayment and use of services (Manning et al. 1984). Persons previously receiving care from fee-for-service physicians were randomly assigned to receive free care from either the Group Health Cooperative of Puget Sound or the fee-for-service physician of their choice. Persons already enrolled at the Group Health Cooperative served as a control group.

The rate of hospital admissions for both groups at the Group Health Cooperative was about 40 percent less than that for the fee-for-service group. Face-to-face visits occurred at the same rate in all three groups, but the number of preventive visits was significantly higher in the two groups in the health cooperative. The expenditure rate for all services was about 25 percent less for persons in the health cooperative than for those in the fee-for-service group. Since population factors were ruled out, the reduced hospital use for patients in the group practice appears to be due to a different style of medicine, one that is much less hospital-intensive and thus less expensive than the medical care provided by fee-for-service physicians.

We conclude from this review that the impact of capitation programs is neither simple nor completely predictable. Even with tight regulatory guidelines, an HMO developer has a good deal of room to maneuver, often in ways that do little to solve the larger problems of efficiency within the system. How successful a particular prepayment structure is in solving these problems may depend as much on its values and its participants' definition of health care as on the structure itself.

CONCLUSIONS

The assessment of performance is just a starting point. From there we can ask whether the health care labyrinth has accomplished its objectives. Should its objectives be changed? What needs to be changed in the way health services are managed? How can such changes best be accomplished? These questions must be pondered within the loosely structured elements of the policy process, or, if you like, the "management subsystem." The assessment of performance does shape the answers to these questions, however. The accomplishments and problems of the health care labyrinth are summarized below.

On the plus side, access to health care has progressively improved since the 1930s. More individuals use more services than ever before. Outcomes, as measured by morbidity and mortality rates, have also improved dramatically. Although they leveled off in the 1950s and early 1960s, mortality and morbidity rates have begun to drop again. Perhaps even more significant has been a narrowing since 1965 of the differences in use of health services, expenditures for health services, and morbidity and mortality rates between lower and higher income groups and white and nonwhite populations.

On the minus side, there are problems concerning the costs of the system. There has been little improvement in productivity to counterbalance the rapid increase in number of units of service delivered and in cost per unit of service. Absorbing these increasing costs, particularly in a period of slow economic growth, is troubling. To paraphrase the song, when the irresistible force of escalating costs meets the immovable object of expenditure limits, something's gotta give.

What will it be? Setting up HMOs does not appear to be a panacea. General structural shifts appear to hold little promise for containing costs without seriously hampering other aspects of performance. We need to search further and dig deeper. In the next section we will look at some of the structural dynamics of the labyrinth. In the final section we will look at ways to escape the existing constraints of the health care labyrinth.

Part
II

Working Within the Labyrinth

4

Organization

Young people today will have
to learn organization the way
their forefathers learned farming.

Peter Drucker

In the first section we described the construction, operation, and performance of the health care labyrinth. In this section we focus on the underlying organizational structures that determine what individual organizations within the system do.

Like any other organizations, organizations in the health care system must reach an accommodation with their environment in order to survive. The environment provides not only the physical resources, such as personnel, funds, and patients, but also the ideological climate that shapes the structure of organizations. Reaching an accommodation with these ideological influences adds to the legitimacy of the organization and helps assure that it will receive the physical resources it needs for survival. In this chapter we explore the implications of the conflicting theories that make up the ideological climate and then describe the process by which organizations adapt to the shifting resources in their environment.

THE IDEOLOGICAL CLIMATE

Individuals create organizations in order to achieve collective goals; they build them according to their ideas of how they can best accomplish these goals. Their ideas may be a naive hodgepodge of conventional wisdom and platitudes, the result of experience in the "real world," or a self-conscious reflection of academic research and theory.

The conflicting assumptions people make about health care and the structures that result from them are summarized in table 4.1. If health care is viewed as an economic good, then it should be subject to the same rules used to produce other economic goods. If, on the other hand, health care is a professional service provided by individuals who have sole command of a socially valued body of knowledge and a socially recognized commitment to provide the highest quality of technical service to all of their patients, then its structure should reflect those objectives. Finally, if health care is a social relationship that is concerned with maximizing the physical and mental well-being of every individual, then a very different structure is required. Once the objective is defined, individuals have a wide array of resources they can call upon to assist in structuring the organization and defending the legitimacy of that structure.

Health Care As an Economic Good

An elegant structure can be built around the definition of health care as an economic good. The health care system becomes a rational organization that produces a product, just as a finely tuned machine might. As described by Max Weber, such an ideal organizational machine, or what he referred to as a "bureaucracy," includes the following basic elements.

1. A clear division of labor exists, and the duties of each office are clearly specified.
2. There is a hierarchy of authority, with each office subject to the discipline of a superior office, but only in terms of the duties of the office—the private life of the official is free from organizational authority.
3. An office holder is an employee; he is a replaceable part and does not personally own his position.
4. Membership in the bureaucracy constitutes a career with distinct ladders and career progression.
5. Hiring and promotion are governed by competence, as measured by training certificates or performance on the job.
6. Impersonality, rather than personal relationships, guides the activities of such organizations (Weber 1947).

Adherence to these principles, which has taken place already in industry in the United States, is becoming increasingly characteristic of health services organizations as well. In fact, a parallel development took place in medicine (Berliner 1984). Rational, or scientific, medicine assumes that all disease is materially generated by specific etiological agents, such as bacteria, genetic malformations, or internal chemical imbalances. Its practice assumes a passive role for the patient and invasive manipulation to restore health. Health, in turn, was increasingly defined as functional capacity, or the ability to perform work (Salmon 1984).

The key to the effectiveness of such a structure is the control it exercises over individual members. There is a clearly defined hierarchy that makes superiors responsible for assuring that the tasks of subordinates are carried out in the prescribed manner. The hierarchy also ties individuals together by providing a clearly defined career ladder up which they can climb, with increasing levels of authority and material reward. Control is further enhanced by the elimination of personal considerations in the recruitment, promotion, and definition of duties of individuals. Who a person's family or friends are should not influence this process. Everything is done by the book—that is, in accordance with objective procedural and personnel manuals.

Such bureaucratic structures have grown in the health sector primarily because they work. For example, the preponderance of opinion and most research suggest that, where medical staff have formulated specific, objective rules concerning admission to and restriction of membership, medical staff performance has been enhanced (Palmer and Reilly 1979, Rhee 1983).

Adherence to a more bureaucratic structure also appears to enhance operating efficiency. For example, lower costs in both medical and nonmedical support departments are reported in hospitals whose administrators and chiefs of staff are knowledgeable about operating statistics and are able to compare their hospital's performance with that of other hospitals in the community. Similarly, a greater number of scheduled meetings among departments and a greater percentage of formal reports prepared and actually sent to the governing board were associated with lower overall costs per case (Shortell, Becker, and Neuhauser 1976).

The logic of the bureaucratic model was refined in the Carnegie steel mills. Fredrick Taylor, author of several influential books on scientific management and the father of modern industrial engineering and operations management, worked in these mills. Managers, he believed, should be "engineers of organizations." He advocated the "scientific" analysis of work and the separation of the planning and organization of work from the performance of it. He believed that designing work in such a way as to incorporate the individual into the larger organization would assure far higher productivity and, since both management and

Table 4.1   **The Conflicting Models (and Ideologies) That Shape the Organization of Health Care Services**

	Model		
	Bureaucratic	Professional	Participatory
Assumption	Health care is an *economic good* subject to the same economic laws as other goods and requiring the same kind of market controls to assure efficient production for consumers	Health care is a *professional service* provided by an elite with sole command of a body of knowledge and with an ethical, socially recognized commitment to provide high-quality service to all consumers	Health care is a *social relationship* that is personal, individualized, and concerned with maximizing the physical and mental well-being of the individual through maximizing his or her sense of control over the accomplishment of these ends
Resulting structure	Duties of individual members clearly specified; clear division of labor based on efficiency	Duties and functions of professionals negotiated with organization; professionals given considerable discretion; more limited, informal division of labor	Open-ended, personal commitments to individuals
	Hierarchy of authority, with each office subjected to the discipline of a higher office, but only with respect to formal organizational functions	Authority based on technical expertise; collegial decision making; disciplining of individual professionals on the basis of personal conduct as well as performance of technical tasks	Egalitarian relationship among participants; collective decision making; no clear boundaries between work and private lives or between clients and providers

Continued

Table 4.1 Continued

	Model		
	Bureaucratic	Professional	Participatory
	A clear career ladder within the organization	Career pursued largely outside the organizational structure; success measured by recognition in the larger professional community rather than position within the organizational hierarchy	No distinction between the career of the individual and the organization—collective achievement
	Recruitment and promotion based on objective evaluation of the individual's ability to further bureaucratic goals	Recruitment and promotion based on personification of professional values, ability to further the profession's goals	Recruitment and promotion based on informal group consensus and personal criteria
	Impersonal—operations based on formal rules; officials' personal values should play no role in decisions and actions	Impersonal—operations based on technical expertise; greater recognition of individual situations; more place for personal (professional) values in the performance of duties	Personal, subjective, and arbitrary; no external, objective criteria for judging actions
Strengths	Stability, efficiency	Adaptability to professional needs; technical quality	Adaptability to individual needs of clients; responsiveness to consumers
Weaknesses	Worker alienation, lack of adaptability	Client alienation, economic inefficiency	Instability, arbitrariness, lack of standards for measuring quality

labor would benefit, would eliminate labor-management conflict. (He was bewildered by the hostility he felt from the workers for his activities in the mills.) Most large health facilities now have industrial engineering departments and use many of the basic principles of scientific management to develop staff, schedule services, and generally attempt to refine procedures to assure greater efficiency. Given the premium that changes in the reimbursement environment have placed on efficiency, industrial engineering is having a greater influence than ever on decisions.

The newfound zeal for scientific management must be tempered with common sense. The approach, initially developed for an uneducated, unskilled immigrant work force, requires far greater collaboration if it is to be effective with the more highly educated work force that exists in most health facilities. Even when economic benefits do materialize, they may not outweigh unanticipated adverse side effects.

> The new administrator of a 200-bed hospital in a small town, concerned with the efficiency of his operation, hired an industrial consulting firm to do an analysis of the hospital's laundry and housekeeping departments. The consultants concluded that, with certain work simplification procedures, the number of employees in both departments could be cut substantially without adverse effects, producing substantial savings for the hospital.

> For a number of years the two departments had provided employment to six mentally handicapped individuals who lived with their families in the community. Even though their pay was minimal, their part in these operations, according to the consultants, did not enhance productivity substantially. Consequently they were among the individuals recommended for firing. Although he was reluctant to do so, the administrator followed the recommendations of the report because he realized that savings would be significant in the long run.

> Upon hearing that they were to be fired, several of the handicapped persons, who had spent all their adult lives working in the institution, collapsed in tears on the floor and could not be consoled. The housekeeping and laundry supervisors were upset; the nurses were upset; several of the doctors were outraged; so was much of the community. The hospital board was equally outraged, and the administrator was fired. All the handicapped employees were rehired. One cannot help feeling that something was missing from the consultants' "scientific" analysis.

There is always the danger that, without constant review, organizations structured around bureaucratic principles can degenerate into caricatures of rational structures, becoming more concerned with form than with substance and with the letter of the law than with the spirit. These perversions, which all of us have seen all too frequently, have transformed "bureaucracy" into a term of derision rather than a standard of organizational rationality.

> State code at the time of construction of the new wing for an institution for the handicapped required that night-lights be constructed in each room two feet below the ceiling. During construction the code was changed, and night-lights had to be placed two feet above the floor. The facility was told to correct these code violations, a process that would be costly. All the patients in this wing, however, were blind (Bicknell 1977).

Health Care As a Professional Service

Defining health care as a professional service creates a different set of expectations about how health services should be structured. If health care is a professional service—that is, if a professional group controls the knowledge and skill necessary to produce that service and undertakes to protect the public's interest—then it should be controlled by the professionals who render that service. In contrast to the bureaucratic approach, the professional approach assumes that certain norms and standards, as well as the basic skills needed to do the job, are internalized by the individual practitioner. Organizations are more decentralized, giving the practitioner a great deal of autonomy. The professional's career is independent of formal organizational structure, and his or her loyalty is to the profession rather than to an organization. A successful professional career involves migrating to progressively more prestigious organizations rather than seeking higher positions within the same organization. Professionals also have more say than bureaucrats in negotiating their role within an organization. There is greater accommodation to the professional's needs than to those of the organization.

The professional approach works best in small organizations that are composed predominantly of fellow professionals. When professionals in larger, more bureaucratic organizations expect a similar degree of autonomy and organizational responsiveness to their needs, they face a serious challenge. There are three tactics commonly used to disrupt the ordinary routines of such structures and force them to be more responsive to professionals' priorities.

Declare a Life-Threatening Emergency. Emergencies and crises ordinarily require circumvention of normal (bureaucratic) rules of operation. For example, carrier-based fighter pilots during World War II were able to ignore most of the rules and protocol of their ships and "requisition" whatever staff and supplies they needed, since at any minute they might be required to go aloft and defend the carrier (Kinzer 1959). Peacetime fighter pilots have been stuck with going through regular channels. Physicians can disrupt the orderly routines of a hospital by declaring a medical emergency. When a patient's life is in danger, the physician can circumvent all the rules and requisition whatever supplies and staff he or she needs. As some observers have noted, physicians have a tendency to label *any* ambiguous event in a hospital as an emergency, thereby claiming the autonomy and responsiveness they want (Freidson 1970, 118).

Invoke a Higher Authority. Organizations gain status, legitimacy, and resources through their ability to accomplish higher goals or values rather than through orderly, efficient operation. Any group that is perceived as being essential to that larger mission, or at least is seen as essential by those in the organization's environment, can call the shots. For example, the test pilots who were recruited to be the first astronauts were initially treated by the engineers and scientists running NASA (the National Aeronautics and Space Administration) in the same way as the chimpanzees that were used on early space flights. After a press conference and a wave of media coverage, the astronauts became closely identified in the public mind with the mission of NASA. Things changed then. United by their new, charismatic media identity, the astronauts were able not only to eliminate some of the more personally aggravating routines, but actually to force the redesign of the space capsule, complete with window (Wolfe 1979).

A hospital would be equally foolish to ignore medical staff concerns about quality of care, even if those concerns seemed more closely related to the staff's own comfort and convenience. For example, unlike other work areas of a hospital, which must make do with canned music, surgical suites are often equipped with stereo tape decks; musical selections are controlled by the surgeon, who feels that the right music helps eliminate the tedium and pressure of surgery and thus assures higher quality outcomes (*New York Times* 1984).

Control the Technology. Emergencies and close identification with the higher mission of an organization can be illusive and transient phenomena. Physicians built medicine, but pilots did not create airplanes

—and knowledge is power. The glamorous fighter pilot's control of the navy bureaucracy in wartime and the astronaut's control of the NASA bureaucracy do not carry over to the commercial airline pilot.

Commercial pilots are subjected to semi-annual physicals, retesting on flight simulators, scrupulous monitoring of their drug and alcohol consumption, and precise delineation of privileges in terms of what aircraft they are allowed to fly. Rigorous training and testing are required before they can fly new, state-of-the-art aircraft. If there is any question about their ability to continue to operate aircraft safely, their commercial license is revoked and they are put out to pasture.

Physicians operate in the wartime fighter pilot mode. Efforts to require relicensure for physicians have lagged far behind even those of other, allied health professions. For all practical purposes, once a physician is licensed, he or she is licensed for life. (The physician does come under some periodic review for hospital privileges, but this does not affect the license to practice.) There are no mandatory periodic assessments of the physician's mental and physical competence, despite the fact that physicians face a far more rapidly changing technology than airline pilots do. Indeed, only one of the medical specialty boards (voluntary certification bodies for medical specialties)—the American Board of Family Practice—now provides for mandatory reexamination. Indeed, there appears to be a general retreat not just from reexamination requirements for physician credentialing, but even from the so-called continuing education requirements, in which few physicians place much faith. (Perhaps the most extreme example of worthless continuing education programs for physicians was a one-week tax-exempt program in Bermuda; the educational sessions consisted of tapes shown while cocktails were served on the flight down.)

Why the discrepancy in control between these two occupations, to both of which the general public entrust their lives? Because *the pilot is the product, not the creator, of the technology.* The physician claims absolute control over the body of knowledge by which his performance may be judged, even though the growing specialization of medicine has strained such a claim and may underlie at least some of the resurgence of interest in more general training. Many observers also believe that the waning interest in reexamination and relicensure is temporary and that pressures from malpractice insurance carriers and increased competition resulting from greater numbers of physicians will stimulate interest and challenge the privileged status of the profession (Weisfeld and Falk 1983, 61–68). Whether this happens or not, physicians, unlike other health professionals, will retain control of the technology and the evaluation of their performance.

Health Care As a Social Relationship

Health care can also be defined as a social relationship. If so, it should be organized differently. Rather than specifying what duties and functions will be performed by each health worker, the structure should emphasize more open-ended personal commitment to patients and to the community in which they live. Rather than setting up a hierarchy of authority based either on position in a bureaucracy or on professional expertise, the structure should encourage more egalitarian relationships among participants and authority based upon consensus. One would expect in such a structure that the boundaries between the roles of providers and clients, and between individual careers and the organization, would become blurred. A decentralized system with relatively small service units and a high degree of client-community ownership would seem to be the structure most compatible with this view of health care.

Such structures, by giving the patient greater control, recognize the critical role the patient plays in the healing process. Evidence suggests that the informal social support provided by such structures is effective in the behavioral and medical management of stress-related disease (Gartner and Riessman 1974) and appears to play a role in producing better health (Asher 1984). Studies have estimated that as many as 90 percent of people who seek medical care are suffering from self-limiting disorders that are well within the body's ability to heal (Fuchs 1974, 64). Many physicians prescribe placebos for patients with such problems and find them surprisingly effective. Some dentists even use what they call "pink pills for pale people," large gelatin capsules full of an inert substance, to relieve the pain experienced by some patients. Why such placebos work was perhaps best explained by Albert Schweitzer, when asked about his close referral relationship with local witch doctors: "The witch doctor succeeds for the same reason all of us succeed. Each patient carries his own doctor inside him. They come to us not knowing that truth. *We are at our best when we give the doctor who resides inside each patient a chance to go to work*" (Cousins 1979, 69; italics added).

There is strong evidence that stress plays a direct role in coronary artery disease, hypertension, ulcers, and stroke, the most common causes of death and disability in the United States. Stress-related suppression of the body's immune system may also be a factor in a variety of other diseases such as pneumonia, influenza, and some forms of cancer (Eyer 1977). The role of an individual's emotional state in such common causes of death and disability as alcoholism, traffic accidents, and suicide is obvious.

The recognition that the individual can prevent illness and heal himself appears to be slowly changing the practice of medicine, as well as that of nursing and other allied health professions. There appears to be greater emphasis on the full participation of patients and families in treatment, more attention to patient education, and greater interest in assisting the patient to deal with the stress-inducing factors in his or her life.

Perhaps the most significant changes have come in the area of chronic care, where no definitive quick fix or curative technology exists. Hospice programs, for example, have demonstrated their cost-effectiveness, thereby winning approval for reimbursement through Medicare. Such programs provide the dying persons greater control over and participation in their care, whether at home or in a home-like setting that substitutes for extended hospitalization. Similar community efforts to coordinate services for the elderly, in lieu of placing them in nursing homes, are promising in controlling some costs and in preventing the mental and physical deterioration that often accompany institutionalization (Mitchell 1978, Doherty, Segal, and Hicks 1978). Efforts are also under way in several states (under court order) to close large state institutions for the mentally retarded and move residents into small, community-based sheltered homes, which appear better able to encourage their development, and at comparable or lower cost.

Even closer to the definition of health care as a social relationship are the self-help movements, aimed at assisting individuals who share common problems associated with an illness. Many involve no economic exchange or professional services at all. Some have been sponsored directly by health care providers to assist their patients. These include zipper clubs (referring to the telltale zipper scar on their chests), which provide mutual assistance for patients recovering from heart surgery, and a variety of support groups for cancer patients. Other self-help efforts have been initiated by patients themselves, unsatisfied with the assistance they received from mainstream medical care. The oldest and largest, Alcoholics Anonymous, has over 750,000 members (Thomsen 1975). It emphasizes peer counseling and intense peer pressure to prevent backsliding (Caplan 1974). Its success in assisting alcoholics has earned it extensive referrals from physicians and the cooperation of most health facilities. Similar self-help programs involving peer counseling have sprung up to deal with such problems as drug addiction, smoking, and weight control. A wide assortment of self-help psychotherapy and mental health support groups has also evolved to fill the needs of their members. They are largely distinguishable by their emphasis on peer counseling and behavioral change rather than on drugs or other forms of medical intervention. They run the gamut from apparently superficial and cynical commercial ventures to very effective programs, such as those mentioned above.

The definition of health care as a social relationship has been most fully elaborated in multidisciplinary therapeutic and educational holistic health centers. There are now approximately 200 such centers in the United States (Gordon 1984). They address the physical, psychological, and spiritual needs of those who come to them for help. Their programs attempt to meet the unique needs of each individual and to mobilize the individual's capacity for self-healing and independence. In practice this has involved placing greater emphasis on client history, client education, and nontraditional therapies such as meditation and biofeedback. Holistic health centers have also generally involved all levels of staff and client volunteers in policy and day-to-day management decisions.

Many health services organizations have tried to adapt their organizational structure to a broader social definition of their mission. Some hospitals, such as Thomas Jefferson in Philadelphia, have moved to a completely decentralized system in which each floor is responsible not only for its own admissions and medical records, but also for its own housekeeping and partial preparation of meals; it has thus avoided many of the foul-ups that plague large teaching hospitals and may have enhanced the quality of the relationship between patients and staff. This reflects a reshaping of hospital organization toward "product-line management," which is now taking place in many institutions. Some hospitals have also implemented primary care nursing, a practice that returns the registered nurse to the bedside and gives him or her responsibility for providing a broad range of services to a small group of patients.

Other health care organizations have moved beyond these relatively minor structural adjustments and have tried, to paraphrase Schweitzer, to give the manager who resides in each employee a chance to go to work. One large HMO network, for example, has instituted a periodic survey to monitor problems perceived by its staff. Information from the surveys has been used to modify referral and consultation procedures and to develop an administrative council to assure greater representation of nonmanagerial personnel in policy formulation (Stebbins, Hawley, and Rose 1982). Some hospitals, borrowing from Japanese industry, have created "quality circles," groups of employees from the same work area who address problems of improved quality and productivity in their area. Such circles meet during regular work hours under the direction of the first-line supervisor, who has received special training in the conduct of such meetings. The circles have generally met with favorable reviews from both employees and managers and have helped solve such problems as excessive overtime among operating-room personnel and excessive nursing staff turnover. While the AHA estimates that about 200 member hospitals are currently experimenting with such programs, there are as yet almost no hard data on their effectiveness (McKinney 1984).

There has been a general resurgence of interest in participatory management (Kuttner 1985). This is due in large part to the striking success of Japanese firms and the relative failure of U.S. automobile and steel firms, long the model for large-scale organization in this country. Japanese firms have a distinctive structure that may account for some of their success (Ouchi 1981). Their strategy appears to be to create an internal culture through which the goals of the organization can be achieved *only* by meeting the needs of the individual members. This strategy produces a peculiar blend of the traditional, paternalistic family enterprise and the modern corporation. It includes the following elements:

— Life-long employment: Individuals enter the organization upon graduation from either secondary school or college and remain in the organization until retirement.

— Nonspecialized career paths: Individuals rotate through many areas, gaining experience in dealing with a broad range of problems.

— Slow evaluation and promotion: Individuals remain for a considerable period of time in a given position before being evaluated and promoted. This encourages managers to focus on conservation and development of the long-term productive, competitive capacity of the organization rather than on short-term largely financial and accounting manipulations that make them appear successful.

— Collective decision making and responsibility: The group is the decision-making unit. Issues are discussed and compromises are made until each individual in the group feels that he or she can support the decision.

— Holistic concern for individuals: The organization's concern goes beyond whether employees are doing their jobs; it includes the individual's family and other activities that may affect performance.

How appropriate are such approaches in the United States? Many of these same themes appear in highly successful American firms. For example, in their best-seller *In Search of Excellence* (1982), Peters and Waterman identify what they believe to be the key characteristics of the most successful corporations in the United States. Considering customers part of the organization's human resources, exhibiting concern for the individual employee, presenting the company as an extended family, and setting up intensive activities to train and socialize personnel are considered critical to high performance. Some of these same principles can be found in failing firms that were turned around after labor began to manage them (Whyte et al. 1983).

There are some remarkable similarities between Japanese firms and health care facilities in the United States (Shortell 1982, Goldsmith 1984). Most hospitals have maintained paternalistic attitudes toward their employees. A large part of the work force in hospitals is made up of women (just as much of the production-level work in some successful Japanese firms is carried out by women). Many of the women who work in hospitals view their employment as temporary, thus assuring hospitals a great deal of flexibility in meeting shifts in demand and financial conditions. It also provides a degree of lifetime job security to other employees (with the possible exception of administrators). Many hospital administrators have specialized backgrounds and were promoted to more general positions, a pattern similar to that in Japanese firms. Collective decision making and responsibility are not foreign to either setting. The major ingredient that appears to be lacking in U.S. hospitals is a comparable financial motivation, and the emergence of DRGs and capitation-based reimbursement mechanisms may well supply this.

Just as there are mock bureaucracies that are irrational, there are mock participatory structures that do not allow participation. While the bureaucratic model limits concern about control over participants to the physical and mechanical aspects of the organization, the participatory approach uses the power of the small informal group and the psychological needs of individuals to achieve its ends. Consequently, a Machiavellian flavor can creep into some participatory management efforts. It is a tribute to the strength of that manager within each individual that these efforts often backfire.

> The key management in a large teaching hospital was concerned about the threat of unionization of nonprofessional employees. Unionization would disrupt the traditional ways of doing things within the institution and infringe on the pre-

rogatives of the top brass. In order to deal with this threat, management hired a group of consultants to run a human relations training course for its supervisory employees. It was hoped that such a program would enable the supervisors to deal more effectively with their employees, reduce dissatisfaction, and therefore reduce the risk of unionization. Since treatment by supervisors had been a source of many employee complaints, the strategy seemed to make sense. Similar institutions had reacted more hysterically to the same threat and had hired, at great expense, public relations firms to engage in crash anti-union campaigns. Their activities had included such innovations as passing out to employees fortune cookies with anti-union slogans inside. The supervisors at the teaching hospital were less concerned with stopping unionization, however, than with stopping the interdepartmental foul-ups that had created animosity among them and with getting what they felt they needed from the top brass. While it is difficult to tell whether they really learned any human relations skills in the class sessions, the sessions did break down their isolation and create a sense of solidarity among them. They began to make militant demands for changes. In the meantime, the nonsupervisory employees voted the union in. The top administrators were then faced with two cohesive, well-organized groups in areas where they had had none. One cannot help feeling it was a healthy development for the institution in the long run.

Accommodating the Models and Ideologies

The perception of health care as an economic good, a professional service, or a social relationship implies a series of choices affecting the structure and operation of a health service organization. If one were to program these choices for a computer, the flow chart might look something like figure 4.1. One would have a clear set of rules for the development and elaboration of organizational structure and clear standards for measuring performance. Further elaboration of the structure would be triggered if performance were unsatisfactory.

The flow chart could even incorporate common adverse consequences of each type of structure. For example, the orderliness of a bureaucracy may make it difficult to adapt to change in the environment and may possibly create alienation among the staff. On the other hand, professional structures can be costly and alienating to patients, and participatory ones tend to be unstable and erratic in their performance.

Figure 4.1 Organizing Health Care Services

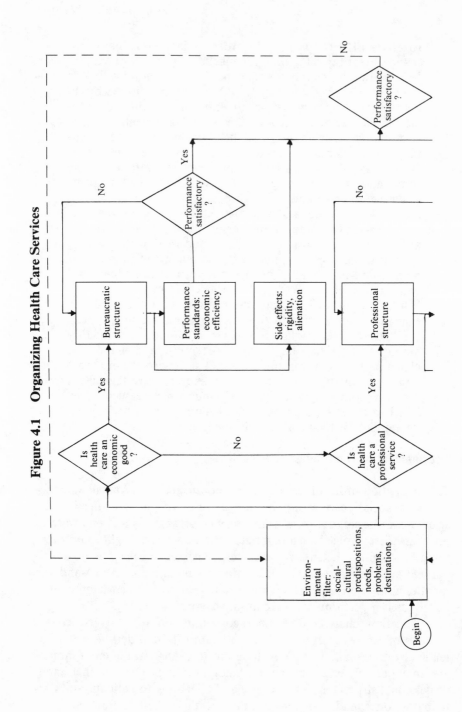

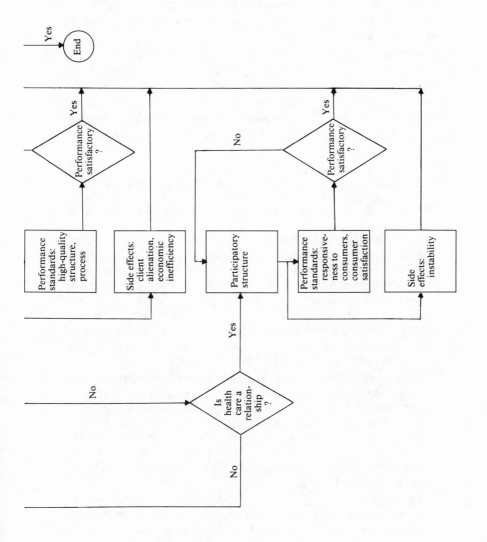

What one would find, however, is that none of these three alternatives would be acceptable. In order for performance to be acceptable, unacceptable side effects would be created. Fortunately, we have a far greater tolerance for ambiguity than computers, and the organizations we create reflect this. In most health care organizations all three assumptions about the nature of the product and the appropriate organizational structure operate simultaneously. In most cases, the ability to absorb such ambiguity and complexity makes for more effective organizations. It also makes for incessant tension about which assumptions and structures will dominate. The argument might go something like this:

> *Bureaucrat*: Health institutions are just like any other large organizations, and the same rules apply. Many people think of bureaucracy as malignant, but the principles that guide it are really the only ones that can make a large organization work. Indeed, the main reason such institutions are not more responsive is that they are not rational. People can get special favors because of personal contacts, and the institutions cannot respond intelligently to the needs of consumers because they are controlled by medieval guilds (professional groups) that resist rational improvements and keep consumers in the dark. Just be careful at whose door you lay the blame for the inefficiencies. If health institutions were really bureaucracies, they would be a hell of a lot more efficient.
>
> *Professional*: You don't know what you're talking about. My obligation is to my patients and I'll give them the best care and treatment my professional judgment and skills can provide. You can't tie my hands. I need autonomy to work most effectively. No rules and regulations will really be effective, since they can never reflect the subtleties of a particular situation or anticipate the exceptions that I must deal with. Give me what I need and get the hell off my back!
>
> *Participatory Advocate*: It matters little to me whether patients are treated as material processed on an assembly line or as cases and diseased organs relegated to detached, cerebral inquiry. Both are equally alienating to patients and nonprofessional workers. They need a sense of control and a sense of involvement and personal worth that neither structure can provide. The key is the quality of the relationship between and among providers and consumers and the degree to which those relationships foster a sense of personal worth and common purpose. Neither the bureaucratic model nor the professional one carried to its logical extreme can pro-

vide this. This can only be achieved with an organizational model that builds in a greater degree of real participation for these individuals.

These arguments will no doubt continue for a long time to come. Health care as a professional service has served as the model for the allied health occupations, and each has struggled to create the same professional immunity that medicine enjoys; each attempts to upgrade training and standards and control entry into its field. Aspiring professionals will attempt to create an enclave within a predominantly bureaucratic structure, transforming what was theoretically a rational structure into an incomprehensible feudal patchwork. It is doubtful that efforts to create independent professional enclaves will be entirely successful in the future, even for physicians; it is equally doubtful that bureaucratic forces will triumph. At best, there will be periodic, uneasy truces between professionals and bureaucrats, truces marred by erratic sniping from individuals attempting to develop more participatory approaches to health care.

DEALING WITH THE ENVIRONMENT

Whatever internal structures are negotiated, the major collective task of an organization is to negotiate an acceptable accommodation with its environment. Organizations, however, do not approach the task in a perfectly rational fashion, even when they have every intention of doing so. An organization tends to divide this task into smaller, more manageable pieces and assign them to different individuals and departments. Time and other resources for solving the problem are limited. As a result, the search for solutions is restricted. It begins with those solutions closest to existing routines and standard operating procedures of the instituion. Solutions that require major disruptions in existing operating procedures and consequently higher risk are avoided. For example, a hospital that needs to work out arrangements for coverage of its emergency rooms will try to come to some agreement with its existing staff before hiring salaried physicians to assure adequate coverage. A hospital interested in expanding its role in ambulatory care will first explore the possibility of constructing a physician office building, giving special preference to existing staff, rather than setting up a separate group practice. A chief of radiology who wants a major new piece of capital equipment, however, may first attempt to get outside donations rather than face the inevitable delays of the internal budgeting process. Organizations and their decision makers, in other words, make choices in terms of what has been called "bounded rationality." They seek solutions that will suffice rather than optimal ones (March and Simon 1964).

An organization follows a set of rules about how it will search for solutions to the problems it encounters (figure 4.2). Failure to achieve acceptable performance at any point triggers further searches for solutions. The organization begins with those searches that have the least invasive implications for it. For example, if a hospital is unable to achieve its desired occupancy levels, its first line defense would be to somehow market its existing activities to increase utilization. If that failed, the hospital would attempt the more difficult and painful task of reappraising its mission and goals and changing itself to fit in better with its environment. This might include closing particular units or changing them to serve patients requiring chronic care. If these efforts fail to increase utilization, the hospital will go out of business, to be replaced by other organizations that are better adapted, through such a process of natural selection, to obtain vital resources. If performance falls within an acceptable range, search activities are shut down and the organization returns to standard, although possibly altered, operating routines. In the remainder of this chapter, we discuss each of these search procedures in more detail.

Search I: Manipulation of the Environment

The first response of any organization to unsatisfactory performance is to attempt to manipulate the environment. Much effort has been devoted to such activities by hospitals in recent years. Marketing, long anathema to physicians, has now come out of the closet. Vice presidents for marketing have become common in hospitals, and marketing activities are being given an increasing amount of administrative attention. Hospitals have engaged in "wellness" campaigns in an attempt to create a favorable public image and to gain a competitive advantage in recruiting private, paying patients. They have advertised in print, on television, and even by sky writing. In the rush of enthusiasm for marketing, some facilities have failed to understand that it involves a good deal more than just attempts to generate demand for existing services: it also means making internal adjustments to respond to unmet demands that facilities are most reluctant to undertake. Some facilities have been guilty of what many people would consider excesses.

Sunrise Hospital's Promotional Program

In the rarefied environment of Las Vegas, Sunrise Hospital, a large proprietary facility, began offering cash rebates for those that would check into the hospital on Fridays and Saturdays. As with most hospitals across the country, occupancy rates drop on weekends. Physicians prefer to stick to a weekday work schedule, and admissions tend to peak on Sunday and Monday and discharges peak on Friday. The promotional program worked. Weekend occupancy rates rose (as did the average length of stay, particularly for elective surgical procedures). The promotional program returned a healthy surplus to the hospital, much to the pleasure of its management—and much to the displeasure of the insurance companies, that refused payments to prevent the continuation of the program. Why? (Intercollegiate Case Clearing House n.d.).

Even relatively straightforward promotional activities for existing services can produce unintended consequences and disrupt internal operating procedures.

The Group Health Cooperative of Puget Sound's Hard Rock Sell

The Puget Sound cooperative in Seattle, Washington, one of the oldest and most respected HMOs, wanted to increase enrollment of young, low-risk subscribers. It was only logical when the newly recruited marketing staff chose the local hard rock music station as their medium and shaped the message accordingly.

"Hey, are you TIRED of SICK CARE? How about joining THE HEALTH CARE plan?" rasped the announcer.

Within hours after the spot was first aired, an eruption equivalent to that of Mount St. Helen's began in the Seattle medical community. The local medical society was enraged by the implication that doctors not in the HMO made people sick. The cooperative's medical staff was enraged by the degradation of having their services offered on a hard rock station (one wonders why so many of them were listening to it). There was concern that the spots would upset the cooperative's efforts to recruit private physicians in outlying communities into a partnership with it and thus seriously hamper efforts to open these new markets. The spot never surfaced again.

Figure 4.2 Organizational Response to Problems in the Environment

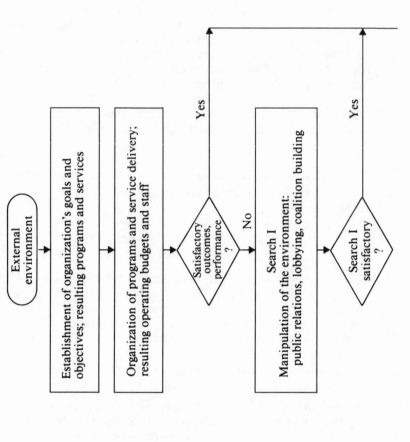

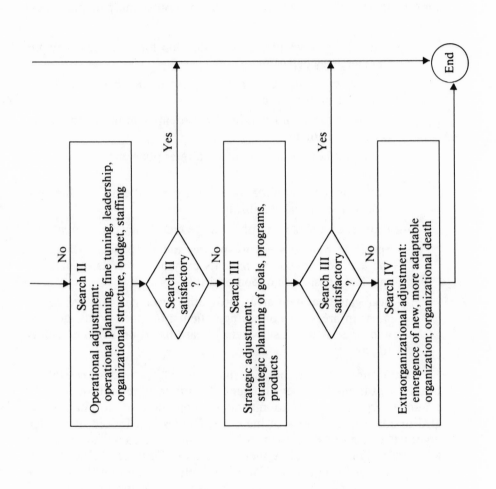

Manipulation of the environment can also mean discouraging utilization. In anticipation of reduced Medicaid funding, the AHA has developed institutional strategies to assure the survival of individual hospitals at the community level (Burns 1981). The report outlines options for "demarketing" services to Medicaid or nonpaying patients. These include:

— Allow lengthy waiting time to develop for nonurgent patients in emergency departments.

— Require cash payment or proof of insurance before rendering service to nonurgent patients.

— Provide little or no parking for patients coming to the emergency department.

— Screen all nonurgent patients and refer poor ones to other providers.

— Transport poor, trauma, or critical care patients to other providers, after initial stabilization.

— Provide an unlisted number for the emergency department.

— Segregate waiting areas for paying and nonpaying patients; in the area for nonpaying patients provide few seats, poor lighting, few signs, and no food or drink.

— Segregate treatment areas, providing fewer staff and less equipment in areas for nonpaying patients; in other words, develop and offer a two-class system of care based on patients' ability to pay.

Environmental manipulation has generally proved successful for health institutions. The development of third-party reimbursement, for example, began with environmental manipulation, as hospitals struggled to adapt to the shock of the Great Depression. Indeed, it is often argued that health care providers have co-opted and used to their own advantage efforts to regulate them externally. Certificate-of-need laws, for example, help moderate, if not eliminate, competition. If there are only enough nursing home or hospital beds in a region to meet needs, full occupancy is guaranteed; further, it is next to impossible to force substandard or hopelessly inefficient facilities to close down (Feder and Scanlon 1980). As a result, patients, particularly those in long-term care facilities, are unable to influence providers through the decisions they make about where they obtain care (Smith 1981). While such controls on supply are aimed at reducing overall cost, they have had little success in achieving this goal (Joskow 1981).

Efforts to shield providers from the cost control pressures of third parties have also met with some success. In general, providers appear to have two responses to state efforts to control or regulate them. First, key staff, accountants, rate setters, and legal counsel are hired to work for either individual institutions or their associations. This tends to ensure a monopoly on knowledge as well as relative inexperience on the regulatory agency's staff. (In one state, for example, a newly formed proprietary nursing home chain hired in one swoop the person responsible for developing the new nursing home Medicaid reimbursement formulas, the head of the state certificate-of-need process, and the supervisor responsible for overseeing compliance with nursing home standards.)

Second, the provider's staff and its technical and financial resources grow dramatically as it enters into full-scale efforts to (1) influence elections, (2) shape the drafting of legislation and regulations, and (3) fight unwanted regulations and legislation in the courts. While providers' interests in regard to regulations and legislation are sharply focused, the public's interests are far broader and more diffuse; hence, legislators and regulators will almost inevitably respond to the providers' more intense pressure (McClure 1981). In general, legislators and regulators are dependent upon the health care industry for information, they lack the resources for a sustained battle with the industry, and they have difficulty absorbing the political costs of decisions that have adverse impacts, such as the bankruptcy of inefficient providers.

In the past, health care organizations have rarely had to look beyond such environmental manipulations to solve their problems. Given the new pressures on the system, however, this situation appears to be changing.

Search II: Operational Adjustment

Failing to achieve satisfactory performance by environmental manipulation, an organization will engage in a variety of internal adjustments in order to improve performance with changing goals and product mix. This is the bread and butter of most managerial jobs. It involves the use of industrial engineering adjustments in staffing and procedures to help improve efficiency and bring performance to acceptable levels. It also involves the use of human relations skills associated with participatory approaches to management. These adjustments need to be sensitive to the environment of a particular unit. The highly developed procedures used for handling the large and predictable volume of appointments in a specialty clinic, for example, will probably be inefficient in dealing with the less predictable demand of a walk-in clinic.

Search III: Strategic Adjustment

Assuming that such operational adjustments fail to bring about acceptable performance, the organization must then undergo some painful soul-searching about its basic structure, objectives, and services. It must adjust its service or product mix in such a way as to assure that the resources it depends upon for its survival—patients, dollars, and skilled medical staff—will be adequate. Hospitals and other providers have become increasingly engaged in strategic diversification, changing both their product mix and their goals to better accommodate themselves to the pressures in their environments, as suggested by the following example.

> In Los Angeles, North Ridge Hospital expects its operating surplus—comparable to a corporation's profit—to increase 12% because it owns, among other things, another hospital; a 73-bed facility to treat alcoholism and drug abuse; a restaurant and shopping center.
>
> In New York, Columbia Presbyterian Hospital hopes to cash in on Manhattan's housing shortage by building condominium apartments.
>
> In Dallas, Baylor University Medical Center owns four hospitals, a construction company, an insurance concern, an office building, a hotel, a health spa and three restaurants. . . .
>
> In Chicago, Lutheran General Hospital sells to employers a preventive-health program that it contends can reduce employee health benefit costs by 15% to 20%. Although the program draws much of its staff knowledge from the hospital itself, it is owned by a separate profit-seeking company which channels revenue back to the hospital in the forms of contributions (*Wall Street Journal* 1981).

Are these the last, desperate acts of drowning organizations, or part of a well-thought-out long-range strategic plan? If the environment is very uncertain, it may not be possible to do effective strategic planning, and long-term survival may depend on the organization's ability to respond quickly to threats and opportunities in its environment. Some organizations, no matter how carefully they plan and adjust their structure, will die; some will survive just by being lucky.

Search IV: Death and Extraorganizational Adjustment

When the three searches fail, an organization dies and whatever it has accumulated in capital assets and goodwill is passed on to its heirs. Such deaths occur regularly. Twenty-five percent of the medical groups operating in 1969 had been disbanded by 1975 (Goodman, Bennett, and Odem 1976, Freshnock and Goodman 1979). Similarly, between 1937 and 1980, 153 not-for-profit acute-care hospitals and 31 public hospitals closed or moved (Sager 1983). Institutional deaths rarely result in the bulldozing of a facility or the conversion of it into condominiums. The most likely heir is a multi-institutional system. These systems now account for 33 percent of all community hospitals (Brown and McCool 1980, Ermann and Gabel 1984, 52). The most striking consolidation has taken place in the proprietary hospital sector. By 1978, the five largest hospital corporations had acquired ownership of 60 percent of all investor-owned hospital beds.

Not all of these mergers, acquisitions, and structural transformations have followed the deaths of organizations. Some have resulted from an organization's own efforts to manipulate its environment and adjust its operations and strategy—efforts to ensure its survival. The reasons that multi-institutional systems are better able to survive will be discussed further in chapter 6. The impact of such transformations on how health care is defined and organized, as we have suggested, is profound.

SUMMARY

Whether health care is considered an economic good, a professional service, or a social relationship implies an underlying ideology and elaborate set of rules concerning how health service organizations should be structured. These ideas or ideologies are only part of the environment to which an organization must adapt in order to assure its survival. An organization will seek to accommodate itself to its environment in whatever way is least disruptive to its existing operations. In the next chapter, we look at how this accommodation affects the organization and its individual members.

5

Individual

All the world's a stage,
And all the men and women merely players.
They have their exits and their entrances,
And one man in his time plays many parts. . . .

William Shakespeare
As You Like It, II, vii

In the previous chapters we described some of the philosophies that
shape the structure of health services organizations and the ways in
which such organizations adapt to their environments. Organizations
are made up of people, however, and people often defy attempts to fit
them into structures. Further, people often subvert efforts to adapt
structures to changes in the environment.

The relationship between people and organizational structure can
be expressed using the theater as a metaphor. In fact, the theater seems
particularly appropriate for institutions so closely associated with the
most intense dramas of life. The perfectly functioning health institution
is like a well-produced theatrical performance: people are carefully selected for each part, the script is rehearsed to perfection, the set is built,
and each scene is performed without a single mistake.

Often, however, each individual actor has developed his or her
own interpretation of his role. In such situations a more appropriate
metaphor would be that of a game. In this chapter we use both meta-
phors to aid in understanding how individuals fit into institutional
structures.

HEALTH CARE INSTITUTIONS AS THEATER

The theatrical metaphor, or role theory, has fallen out of favor as a method of analyzing organizational problems. It is not a rigorous research tool; nevertheless, it is a viewpoint that can be valuable in sorting out some of the problems that occur between individuals and the organizations they inhabit. An acquaintance with some of the basic terminology of role theory is necessary to this analysis.

Role

Role refers to the conduct associated with a certain position or part rather than with the player who recites the lines or performs the prescribed function. Roles are the building blocks of both theatrical productions and organizations. They serve to link an individual's activities to the activities of others and to those of the organization (Katz and Kahn 1978, Roos and Starke 1981).

Role Set

Roles are located within a network of other parts or positions with which the role player, or *focal person*, must interact. This network, or *role set*, influences the way the actor plays his or her part, just as relevant organizations in a health agency's *organization set* influence its behavior. Figure 5.1 illustrates that the nurse must contend with pressure from nursing supervisors, hospital administrators, physicians, patients, other nursing staff, and the professional associations to which he or she belongs. Similarly, the director of a health care business coalition's role is shaped by his or her board members, other staff, and the expectations of the institutions and third parties with which the director must deal.

Each member of the role set attempts to influence the behavior of the focal person. All roles have a certain amount of ambiguity; as a result, the persons who occupy a particular role often face conflicting expectations. These ambiguities and conflicts may be resolved through negotiations between the focal person and the other members of his or her role set. Through this process, the focal person's concept of his or her role and the expectations of the people with whom he or she deals may be brought closer together. The give-and-take that results is essential to the effective operation of a health care institution.

**Figure 5.1 Role Sets for the Urban Nurse and
Director of a Health Care Business Coalition**

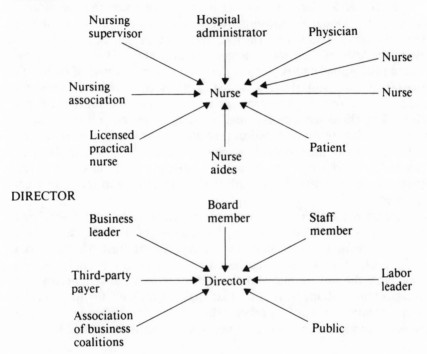

Role Conflict

The negotiating process is rarely a smooth one. Great diplomacy may
be required. Destructive confrontations can occur when *role senders* do
not communicate their expectations clearly enough to the focal person.
Often role senders communicate their expectations indirectly, through
subtle signals such as raised eyebrows, a cough, or an offhand comment.
Not all actors are adept at picking up these cues; some may even be unaware of the cumulative effects of these cues on their behavior. No matter what the particular style of communication and no matter what the
ability of the actor to perceive that communication, the cumulative impact may be difficult for the focal person to avoid or to handle. The resulting role conflict can produce, in extreme forms, psychological disor-

ders for the individual and chaos for the organization. The sources of such conflict are perhaps easier to identify than to alleviate (Katz and Kahn 1978).

Person-Role Conflict. Conflict is inevitable when the characteristics of an individual are incompatible with the requirements of the role he or she plays. The Peter Principle, which holds that people routinely rise to the level of their incompetence, is alive and well in most health-related institutions and is perhaps the most common cause of such conflict (Peter and Hull 1967). Often the only way to reward competent technical performance is to promote an individual to a supervisory position. The characteristics essential to being an effective nurse, laboratory technician, or other technical specialist, however, may be irrelevant to being a good supervisor. Consequently the common complaint is, You lose a good nurse (or whatever) and gain a poor supervisor. The transition can be difficult for both the organization and the individual involved.

Perhaps a more concrete example of person-role conflict—and one that presents a problem in many hospitals—occurs in the case of the young, professional status-conscious female nutritionist who is placed in the position of supervising the embittered, inner-city male kitchen help. Both the nutritionist and the kitchen help have stereotypes and preconceptions about their roles that make it difficult for them to develop an effective working relationship. Sporadic warfare ensues, and outside intervention may even be necessary to settle the squabbles.

Intersender Conflict. *Intersender conflict* occurs when two or more role senders have conflicting expectations. Nurses and medical record librarians often find themselves in situations where administrative (bureaucratic) controls and routines conflict with a physician's demands.

Planners face similar problems. Some local board members still see the health planning agencies as vehicles for gaining the additional health services their communities want. The health planning agencies, however, are evaluated at the federal level on the basis of their ability to control costs, and they are expected to limit the expansion of services in their region.

Novices find these conflicts difficult to handle, whereas more experienced persons have developed mechanisms for coping with them. Nurses who have worked longer at a given hospital tend to report fewer problems in dealing with the conflicting demands of physicians, patients, and administrators than do nurses with less experience (Smith 1970).

Intersender role conflict is particularly acute in health care institutions—not simply because of the multiple lines of authority that exist there, but also because there is often little agreement among role senders as to the nature and scope of their own and others' authority. One study of "interprofessional teamwork" between physicians and nurses concluded that there was so little agreement about role expectations that the concept was meaningless (Temkin-Greener 1983). Their differing expectations represented basic philosophical differences rather than simple misunderstandings that could be cleared up with adequate communication.

Inter-role Conflict. *Inter-role conflict* occurs when the expectations surrounding one role an individual plays are in conflict with those surrounding another role that individual plays. Professional and family roles, for example, are often hard to integrate, and the transition between the two is not easy.

Inter-role conflict can be present even when the activities are similar. Consider, for example, the supervisory nurse who is active in a state nursing association that is involved in quasi collective bargaining with hospitals. Demands from the state association require aggressive leadership for pay increases, but these conflict directly with pressures from administrative colleagues within the hospital to keep nursing costs at a minimum. In many areas of the hospital, supervisory roles are combined with the work performed by subordinates. Thus a person may play the role of both colleague and supervisor, a situation that often leads to inter-role conflict.

Intrasender Conflict. When contradictory messages come from the same source, the result is *intrasender conflict*. Personnel within an admitting office might be instructed to be considerate and sensitive to individual needs and problems; at the same time, they are reminded of the necessity of obtaining financial information before admitting a patient to the hospital. The problem arises when an admissions clerk encounters a seriously injured patient. The clerk must then decide between obtaining the needed financial information and waiving the normal procedure.

Intrarole Conflict. The individual's role may have built-in contradictions. For example, most contacts with patients involve both the performance of mechanical technical tasks and the provision of emotional support and reassurance. These aspects are not easy to combine, and the result is that there is always a certain amount of tension between the two. Nurses tend to perform more of the supportive (expressive) function, and physicians tend to perform more of the technical (instrumental) function, although both their roles require each (Johnson and Martin 1958). In addition, although both roles require that the individual be warm and supportive to the patient, a certain amount of emotional detachment (affective neutrality) is also required. Warm, cordial relationships are appropriate, but close, personal ones are not. It is often difficult to make such distinctions, however.

Role Overload. Often there are simply too many external and internal expectations for an individual to handle. The doctor who sees 60 patients a day, the nurse who is responsible for 20 surgical patients, and the administrator whose time is spent putting out fires are all likely to suffer from role overload. Common symptoms are irritability, cynicism, and emotional exhaustion.

It is often difficult to accept limitations on what one can do. The expectations of patients, the public, and one's colleagues can make it hard to cope with failure. Often expectations and reality are too far apart.

What If There Is No Cure?

I do feel awful now.

Have we not just sent men to the moon? To the deep ocean floor? Do we not transplant hearts and grow babies in test tubes and decode the double helix of life? Has not a living baby been born from a mother six days dead? Is there not hope of computerizing genetics? Then why should anything at all be beyond fixing?

That is just how patients approach us: fix it, you pompous, inflated guardian of special techniques, for we know that *everything* can be fixed. If you fail, you shall be taken to task —and perhaps to court—for your incompetence.

That is just how residents approach us: teach us how to fix it, for we have been promised that *everything* can be fixed, and we shall be bitterly angry and disappointed if you fail us (Lederer 1970, 30–31).

There is a variety of defense mechanisms that individuals, with the help of bureaucratic and professional structures, can use to avoid coping with or facing such issues. In the case of nurses, such defense mechanisms may involve disengagement and the displacement of energies elsewhere.

Generally a nurse confronted with a hopeless case finds it easiest to maintain her composure when the patient can be made comfortable with sedation and a minimum of talk. Nurses will often ask doctors for flexible sedation orders so they can control the dosage; and occasionally may even give the patient more sedation than either he or the doctor wants. They can be considerate and attentive, and yet confine themselves only to the patient's existence as a medical problem, a body (that is, socially dead).

Nurses do have standard tactics for avoiding upset when a patient—especially one with strong appeal, like an attractive child—dies or is dying. They "switch objects" if they can—concentrate intensely on some other patient for whom there is still hope, and let someone else, a chaplain perhaps, take over the death watch. They try to minimize the loss—the patient could not have led a normal life, death stopped his suffering, he died easy of mind because he left his family well fixed. They speak of God's will. They try to absolve themselves of negligence and believe they did all they could. They try various kinds of catharses—crying, talking, keeping busy. Most important, they try to forget—or at least block the memory off: "We talk over death here, get our feelings out, then forget it and go home."

Are these methods always desirable? Perhaps not—no methods are always desirable. But maintaining composure and efficiency are more than matters of personal comfort or expressions of hardheartedness. Death takes no holiday. The next patient coming up from emergency may also need competent, steady care and solace on the passage out (Glaser and Strauss 1970, 141–42).

Another defense is to deny the importance of an event and treat it with exaggerated casualness. This occurs in the case of emergency room physicians faced with possible DOAs (persons dead on arrival), which are signalled in advance by ambulance sirens.

In nearly all DOA cases the pronouncing physician (commonly that physician who is the first to answer the clerk's page or spot the incoming ambulance) shows in his general demeanor and approach to the task little more than passing interest in the event's possible occurrence and the patient's biographical and medical circumstances. He responds to the clerk's call, conducts his examination, and leaves the room once he has made the necessary official gesture to an attending nurse. (The term "kaput," murmured in differing degrees of audibility depending upon the hour and his state of awakeness, is a frequently employed announcement.) It happened on numerous occasions, especially during the midnight to eight shift, that a physician was interrupted during a coffee break to pronounce a DOA and returned to his colleagues in the canteen with, as an account of his absence, some version of "Oh, it was nothing but a DOA."

It is interesting to note that, while the special siren alarm is intended to mobilize quick response on the part of the emergency room staff, it occasionally operated in the opposite fashion. Some emergency room staff came to regard the fact of a DOA as decided in advance; they exhibited a degree of nonchalance in answering the siren or page, taking it that the "possible DOA" most likely is "D." In so doing, they in effect gave authorization to the ambulance driver to make such assessments. Given the time lapse which sometimes occurs between that point at which the doctor knows of the arrival and the time he gets to the patient's side, it is not inconceivable that in several instances patients who might have been revived died during this interim. This is particularly likely in that, apparently, a matter of moments may differentiate the revivable state from the irreversible one (Sudnow 1970, 113–14).

Resolving Role Conflict

The structure of an organization can create conflict. Less structured wards, for example, provide individuals and groups with greater flexibility; this flexibility can lead to greater role uncertainty but less person-role conflict than more structured situations (Palola and Jones 1965). Attempts to clarify roles with written procedures and regulations often result in even more conflict because of differing interpretations. Since no written procedures can possibly anticipate all situations a particular employee will face, the most effective form of sabotage possible in a health-related institution would be for an employee or group of employees to stick rigidly to written procedures.

Because role conflicts can never be completely resolved, efforts to lessen them tend either to minimize the need for give and take between roles or to create an environment that will facilitate give and take. Well-defined jobs are not enough: individuals must somehow be insulated from persons who make conflicting demands on them and have conflicting perceptions of them. This is suggested in the classic solution developed for waitresses and hospital laundry workers.

Is Communication Really Necessary?

The human relations tradition and the organizational developers who inherited it stress the need for effective communication between various groups. Yet when conflicting status and orientations are involved, this is not necessarily a good idea. For example, industrial corporations have found it useful to segregate research and development activities from production, even locating such activities in different sections of the country.

A classic human relations problem was highlighted in a study of the restaurant industry. Waitresses found themselves caught between the conflicting demands of high-status male customers and a high-status and often temperamental male chef. As a result, morale was low and absenteeism and turnover high. The solution adopted was not to work toward better communication between the waitresses and the chef, but instead to minimize contact between them. A pass-through spindle system was installed; this allowed the waitresses to place orders without confronting the chef. Similarly, the chef used a pass-through shelf to fill orders and thus did not have any contact with the waitresses. Due to these changes, morale among waitresses improved, as did the stability of the work force (Whyte 1948).

Laundry workers in hospitals enjoy an insulation similar to that created for waitresses by the spindles. Though their work is hot, smelly, dirty, and repetitive, laundry department employees almost invariably have far lower turnover and absenteeism rates than employees in other, comparable departments in the hospital. For example, there is much higher absenteeism and turnover in the housekeeping and dietary sections, even though wages are comparable and the physical surroundings more pleasant. The only explanation for this difference seems to be that the laundry workers are isolated from high-status groups in the hospital. They usually work in a small, compact setting that allows a good deal of interaction with fellow workers and minimum harassment from outsiders.

The alternative to isolating workers from the conflicting demands of others is to create situations that will promote interaction and improve the role-sending and role-taking ability of those involved. Many management strategies advocated in the popular literature make use of role theory. One such strategy, management by objectives, is simply a formalized attempt to legitimate and facilitate role negotiation. In hospitals, process consultation and most other techniques of organizational development are largely geared to the process of role taking and sending and to facilitating that communication process. One intervention to enhance communication provided nursing supervisors with greater feedback from their subordinates; this produced practices that provided more open expression of views and joint problem solving. This, in turn, led to reduced reports of role conflict, ambiguity, and stress among nurses. Job satisfaction was increased and absenteeism reduced (Gray-Toft and Anderson 1985).

How people perceive different role demands will determine how willing they are to act upon them. Consider the following scripts:

Role Negotiation in an Urban Hospital

Assistant Administrator: You know the financial pressures we're under. Cutting the dietary staff and letting the nurses distribute the food trays is one of the only ways we can cut corners without further reducing nurse staffing.

Director of Nursing: I objected to the whole thing from the beginning. How can you expect skilled professional nurses to perform such functions? Now look what's happened. We're facing a walkout. The nurses refuse to do it. They say it's not nursing. They've got backing from the state nursing association. This is a crisis situation. If we don't back off, the whole roof's going to cave in. We've lost some of our best ones already.

Role Negotiation in a Suburban Hospital

Director of Nursing: We've been talking it over in the new unit. You've got to get those dietary aides off the floors. The nurses should really be the ones to give the food trays to the patients; it's an important part of our function. We need to have some more pleasant ways of interacting with patients so we can develop a better, more supportive relationship with them. Some of the patients really shrink every time we come into their rooms. They know that all we're going to do is force some medicine down their throats or give them an injection. It's important for nurses to be able to keep track of what patients are eating.

Assistant Administrator: I can understand how you feel about it. There may be some problems working it out with the dietary department, but I'll see what I can do.

In order to understand these episodes, one has to understand the factors that shaped the situations. One has to take into account the characteristics of the organizations and of the persons involved as well as the interpersonal dynamics. The large urban teaching hospital is faced with serious deficits and nurse-to-patient ratios that are tight in comparison with other kinds of hospitals. There is little financial lee-way to do the kinds of things the administration would like to do in the large, impersonal units in that hospital. The suburban hospital, on the other hand, is operating with a comfortable surplus. It is a new facility, with small, circular units and a relatively high staff-to-patient ratio.

The nurses in the two settings are also quite different. Those in the urban medical center are younger, more highly trained, and consider themselves specialists in the care of particular kinds of patients. They see the route to professional advancement as following the medical model toward specialization and greater involvement in the technical care and treatment of patients. The nurses in the smaller, suburban hos-pital are somewhat older and less self-consciously concerned with their profession or with mastering new skills.

There are also clear differences between the interpersonal events surrounding each of these episodes. The imposition of a new task by someone not only from outside the work group but also from outside the professional reference group is quite different from an internally ini-tiated negotiation with an outsider for a change in responsibility. Be-cause of these differences, one situation becomes a knock-down-drag-out confrontation over the power of a professional group to determine the work it will do, while the other is a negotiation with a professional group whose power seems to be taken for granted.

The Plot

Role conflicts make good drama. In health care settings there is a stan-dard plot to such dramas that one sees again and again. In simplest terms, the plot involves a struggle to define what health care is and, consequently, what health organizations and the individuals who work within them should be doing.

Both the institutions and the individuals involved suffer from multiple personalities. Health care can be an economic good, a profes-sional service, or a social relationship. Each implies a somewhat differ-ent organizational structure and different role expectations for the participants.

The standard plot for role conflicts in health settings can be seen in the two scripts about who was to provide food for patients. The administrator in the urban hospital saw health care as an economic good that could be organized rationally, while the director of nursing saw it as a professional service. The director of nursing in the suburban hospital defined health care as a personal relationship with patients.

The bureaucratic model tends to predominate in the routine, hotel-type services within a health care institution. The professional model is realized most nearly by physicians, while patients' roles often match the participatory model.

HEALTH CARE INSTITUTIONS AS GAMES: TRANSACTIONAL ANALYSIS

The theatrical metaphor is of little help in explaining how competing bureaucratic, professional, and participatory role expectations are actually resolved. Organizational life in health care settings is not as orderly and predictable as the theatrical metaphor implies. It is probably more accurate to look at it as an elaborate, chaotic series of games rather than as a well-produced and well-directed theatrical production.

Eric Berne in *Games People Play* (1964) has provided the clearest framework for understanding the process. His book provided a popularized synthesis of role theory and more traditional psychoanalytic thought. According to Berne, games are part of a hierarchy of social interactions in which individuals engage. Social interaction derives from basic human needs for stimulation, recognition, and structure. We require stimulation from others, and we need a certain amount of recognition in order to maintain our psychological equilibrium. We also need to structure these social transactions so that we know what to do and what to expect from others. Thus, in order of increasing complexity, these transactions may take the form of rituals, activity, pastimes, games, and intimacy. In addition, each transaction takes place somewhere along a continuum from complete social withdrawal to intimacy. The position of a transaction along that continuum indicates both the seriousness of the personal commitment involved and the complexity of the interaction.

Rituals are the simplest form of social activity. A ritual is a stereotyped series of simple complementary transactions programmed by external social forces (Berne 1964, 36). They may be formalized into institutional rituals, such as those that make up a great deal of the contact between a patient and members of a hospital staff. Through such rituals staff members routinely meet those parts of their formal job assignments that call for social contact with patients. These requirements may also be met through informal rituals, such as those involved in the following exchange:

Aide: Hi!
Patient: Hi!
Aide: How are you feeling today?
Patient: Fine. Is the weather hot enough for ya?
Aide: Yup. Hope it cools off tomorrow.
Patient: Well, take care.
Aide: So long.
Patient: So long.

Berne refers to such a ritual as stroking. No real information is exchanged, and only limited ritualistic recognition is given the other person. The amount of stroking required depends on the depth of our acquaintance with another individual. The more closely acquainted they are, the more stroking will be mutually required before two individuals can get down to the business that brought them together.

Activity involves "simple, complementary, adult transactions" (Berne 1963, 147). The terse, direct communication between the various actors in a surgical suite as well as most other transactions involving the accomplishment of a common task fall into this category. Yet, no matter how structured the work, there is always plenty of time for pastimes and games.

Pastimes are "a series of semi-ritualistic, simple, complementary transactions arranged around a single field of material, whose primary object is to structure an interval of time" (Berne 1964, 41). Such activity takes up most of the time at social gatherings, whether at professional meetings or more informal gatherings. It concerns reminiscing about past experiences ("Remember when? . . ."), friends ("Whatever happened to? . . ."), and possessions ("How do you like your new? . . ."). It provides a pleasant way of filling time.

A *game* is "an ongoing series of complementary ulterior transactions progressing to a well-defined, predictable outcome" (Berne 1964, 48). Unlike rituals and pastimes, games involve ulterior motives and are essentially dishonest. They involve a kind of dramatic payoff not found in either rituals or pastimes, and they may be an inevitable fixture of organizational life. Some theorizing has called into question the value of looking at organizations as entities in themselves with goals and objectives of their own (Weick 1969). Perhaps it would be more useful to view organizations as a series of multiparty games involving shifting coalitions that attempt to control the distribution of resources within the organization. Organizational goals, then, are a reflection of these shifting, competing influences and cannot be separated from the actors involved.

Intimacy involves a "direct expression of meaningful emotions between two individuals without ulterior motives or reservations" (Berne 1963, 148). Such transactions have a place within the participatory conception of organizations but are unlikely to occur in either bureaucratic or professional conceptions. Those involved in such transactions in either bureaucratic or professional structures are probably violating requirements for impersonality and risk being accused of either nepotism, favoritism, or unprofessional conduct.

Organizational Transactions

Berne argues that there are three kinds of ego states, or states of mind, through which an individual can enter into transactions:

1. Those that resemble the ego state of a parent, that is, of someone acting parentally
2. Those in which facts offered by the environment are dealt with objectively
3. Archaic ego states that resemble closely those found in infants and children of various ages (Berne 1963, 163)

Berne refers to these three states as parent, adult, and child. He views the child as a relic of the behavior, attitudes, and feelings of the individual's own childhood. The parent ego state is usually stimulated by the childlike behavior of another and may be either nurturing or dogmatic and disapproving. It, too, is a relic of an individual's past experience and often reflects the orientation of influential parental figures in one's own life. The advantage of the parent state is that it makes many of an individual's decisions automatic: since the parent treats new situations in terms of behavior that was prescribed in the past, he need not subject himself to prolonged or agonized questioning. The adult is an independent set of feelings, attitudes, and behavior adapted to current reality and unencumbered by leftover childhood or parental responses.

As a tool for organizational analysis, and particularly for analysis of health care organizations, Berne's framework requires certain elaboration and alteration. His concepts of the parent, adult, and child need to be merged with the organizational models. We want to avoid making any value judgments about which ego state is preferable for an organization—what may be good for an individual is not necessarily good for an organization, and which model is appropriate depends upon its collective purpose.

Basically there are three orientations, or states of mind, that one can adopt in relationships with organizations: *child-participant, adult-professional,* or *parent-bureaucrat.*

The Child-Participant Orientation. Few people are born into large, formal, impersonal organizations; those who are often have to pay heavy psychic costs. The family environment that presumably provides the best conditions for a growing child is quite different from a formal bureaucratic structure. Such families provide a good deal of warmth, affection, nurturing support, and opportunity for personal growth. Spontaneity is valued, and interactions among members are largely an end in themselves. Formal rules are minimized, and what structure exists is more a cooperative, collaborative one than an externally imposed, authoritarian one. This description seems to characterize accurately the lost tribe of Stone Age people discovered in the Philippines as well as the fantasies of Rousseau, John Stuart Mill, and modern adhocracies suggested by Toffler (1969) and Mintzberg (1983). All place a value on spontaneity and creativity in organizations, and all see their basic purpose as mutual nurturance.

Everyone has a bit of this orientation. One tends to resist formal structure, performance evaluation, and external controls. One would like to treat other persons as whole and uniquely valuable human beings and be treated by them in the same way. Many persons attracted to health careers appear to have a stronger child-participant orientation than others do.

When physicians, nurses, and administrators are asked why they chose their respective careers, the answer given most frequently is that they seemed to provide an opportunity to work with and help people. Physicians also tend to report an attraction to the personal independence and autonomy promised by a medical career as opposed to careers pursued within large bureaucratic settings (Bucher and Stelling 1977). Other occupational groups in the health sector with professional aspirations seem to share this perspective.

The Adult-Professional Orientation. The education or training one receives creates a different orientation. One learns that objective knowledge and expertise are the source of authority and that decisions should be made on the basis of objective evidence rather than personal considerations or organizational tradition. Allegiance to a specific organization is limited. One's real identity lies with one's professional group, which operates independently of formal organizational boundaries. Such an individual expects to negotiate his role within an organization rather than have it dictated to him. He expects a good deal of say in what he does and how organizes his work. He is, after all, an adult (professional).

It is not surprising that Berne, a physician by training, sees this as the most desirable state of mind. Because of their professional status, physicians are able to adopt this orientation toward the organizations they work in with relative ease. However, when dealing with other groups, such as nurses, physicians assume parental patterns of authority and control and force others to assume more passive, childlike positions (Freidson 1970).

The Parent-Bureaucrat Orientation. To the extent that one identifies with the standard operating procedures and routines of a large, formal organization, one has adopted the parental, or bureaucratic, orientation. One is concerned not so much with whether a particular procedure makes sense, but with whether it is "the way we do things here." The rules are viewed as guides to conduct, and the parent-bureaucrat wants procedures nailed down in writing. A strict hierarchy of authority, a narrow division of labor, and an externally formalized prescription of role behavior are seen as the way to run an organization effectively.

Each of these orientations implies different organizational structures. There is a bit of the child, professional, and bureaucrat in every organization, just as there is in the individuals who make them up. People with a particular orientation will struggle to impose that orientation on the institution, or they may even assume that the institution already operates on the basis of that orientation. Sufficient role insulation will assure that they will never discover otherwise.

Many of the transactions that take place in organizations are games that reflect these orientations and subsequent attempts to shape the institution. We will look at some of these games for illustrative purposes.

Complementary Transactions As Games

Complementary transactions are those in which both parties understand and accept their roles and the ground rules that surround their transactions. Some of the most typical complementary transactions are shown in figure 5.2 (as is the convention with this kind of scheme, the arrows pointing from right to left represent the other's response). The four pairs of arrows in figure 5.2 complement each other, thus stable, predictable transactions are possible.

The simplest games are probably those that involve parent-parent, adult-adult, or child-child transactions. These games involve manipulating the other party within the ground rules of a bureaucratic, profes-

Figure 5.2   Typical Complementary Transactions

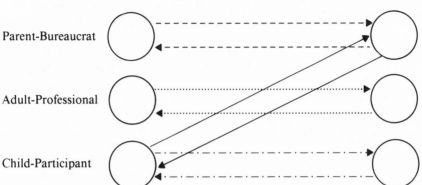

Parent-Bureaucrat

Adult-Professional

Child-Participant

Adapted from: Berne, Eric. 1964. *Games People Play.* New York: Random House, p. 32. Copyright © 1964. Reprinted by permission.

sional, or participatory framework. The game may be one in which one party wins and the other loses, or it may be an additive game in which both sides can win by scoring points.

One can conceive of *parent-parent* games being played between a hospital administrator and a Blue Cross representative negotiating rate increases for the hospital. Both parties accept the essentially bureaucratic process, and consequently their transactions focus on how the procedures work and what is permissible within the rules that govern the process. The rules are unquestioned, even though some may be absurd or without relevance for the particular situation that the hospital faces. Nevertheless, both the administrator and the Blue Cross representative understand their parental roles, and they maneuver within those constraints. In fact, the rules may be so ingrained that the individuals do not even question them subconsciously.

Adult-adult transactions are more questioning, factual, and objective. They are illustrated by the transactions involved in rounds in a teaching hospital. While at one level these transactions provide an adult problem-solving activity, oneupmanship also enters in as the participants try to match wits.

Rounds

On the morning after a patient's admission, during "work rounds" from 7:45 to 9:00, when the ward team goes from patient to patient, the student is expected to summarize informally the history, physical, and lab tests for the benefit of those team members who were off duty the previous night. A formal discussion is given by the student during "visit rounds" later in the day, when he relates the details of the case to the visiting physician, usually just called "the visit." The visit is a staff member of the hospital, assigned to the wards for a month, and legally responsible for all the patients on the ward.

The student's formal discussion is known as "presenting." To present a patient means to deliver the salient information in a brief, highly stylized form. The student is expected to do this from memory. A presentation begins with events leading up to admission for the present illness; then goes on to past medical history; then a review of organ systems; family and social history; physical findings beginning at the head and working down to the feet. Laboratory data is then presented in a specific order: blood studies, urine studies, cardiogram, X-rays, and finally more specialized tests.

The entire process is not supposed to take more than five minutes.

A good presentation is difficult, for along with summarizing positive feelings, the student is expected to include certain "pertinent negatives" from among the almost infinite number of symptoms and signs the patient does *not* have. These pertinent negatives are intended to exclude specific diagnoses. Thus, if a patient has jaundice and a large liver, the student should state that the patient does not drink, if this is the case.

Aggressive students can be quite abstruse in their negatives, hoping that the instructor will interrupt and ask (for example): "What were you thinking when you said the patient had never danced in Tibet?"

To this the student can triumphantly name some obscure disease that vaguely fits the situation, such as "the Kurelu Dancing Syndrome, sir." He thus appears well-read. The game can be dangerous with a knowledgeable visit, however, for he is likely to shoot back: "The Kurelu Dancing Syndrome never occurs in males under forty, and your patient is thirty-six. If you want to do some reading, I refer you the *Kurelu Medical Journal*, volume ten, number two." This is a signal for the student to crumble; he has lost the round—unless, of course, he has a rejoinder. There is only one acceptable form: "But, sir, in the *Mauritanian Journal of Midwifery* last week there was a report of a case in a ten-year-old boy." This may, or may not, work. The visit may reply, "The *what* journal? Wasn't that the one which reported that skimmed milk caused cancer?"

That ends the discussion (Crichton 1970, 174–76).

Child-child complementary transactions involve more emotional, subjective interchanges. The stakes in games involving such transactions are more personal and emotional than the professional and bureaucratic stakes of parent-parent and adult-adult games.

Laughter in the Ward

Although some patients are more gifted than others in highlighting the "comic element" of their experiences, most of them, when sitting together in the television room or conversing in the ward, tend to fall into jocular conversation.

Here is a sample of conversation in the television room: "Did you hear what happened yesterday? I'm telling yah, it was a riot. The funniest thing!"

The story is then told of the mixup between two Mrs. Ann Broseman's, which resulted in the wrong one, poor Mrs. Broseman from the medical ward, being taken from the TV room by an intern from the surgical ward and being subjected to an elaborate physical examination in the surgical ward.

In the meantime, the nurses in the medical ward were looking for Mrs. Broseman. They were all excited and worried because they *are* responsible for the patients, you know. Well, finally, they got her. She was raving and red as a beet. She came here for high blood pressure in the first place. Well, it must have gone sky-high after that!

This incident touches on certain threatening aspects of hospital life, for there are fears, common to all, that some confusion in administering medication might occur. But by making the story seem funny, the storyteller implies that even if such fears were realized, even if the confusion occurred, it would have ridiculous rather than disastrous consequences. And the ridiculous victim ("red as a beet"), damaged in dignity but not in body, proves that those fears were groundless.

This story also channels and releases hostility against the nurses and introduces a comic reversal of roles. It is the nurses, not the patients, who are "excited and worried." Such a reversal of roles is a frequent element in comic representations.

Jocular talk not only reassures, it also socializes in other ways. Jocular griping transforms socially inadmissable complaints into approved forms of striking back at ward routine. It helps both the complainer and his listeners to come to terms with their condition and with ward life. "I never complain," one patient said. "What good would it be anyhow? No use complaining. . . . Got to take things as they are. Take life as it is. Some people magnify things. Others make them smaller. That's the better way." In her jocular talk to other patients, this patient "made things smaller" not only for herself but for the other patients as well (Coser 1962, 84–85).

The excited, childlike talk and griping on the ward entertains the patients and creates a sense of cohesiveness among them that helps to make their experience a little less lonely and frightening. Patients often tend to see the physician as a protecting parent, and they tend to evaluate his performance on that basis. When asked, "How would you describe a good doctor?" patients typically respond:

"The main thing: talks nice to me. Gives me hope. Some doctors will come in and give prescriptions and run out."

"When the doctor takes interest. . . . Some doctors, they come in and don't look at you."

"One who knows what he is doing . . . who is sociable; some come in and don't talk."

"If he considers his patient and doesn't rush him to go home."

"He is not too good a doctor. He is a mechanic. He is a Harvard graduate . . . gave me a speech and that's all. . . . There was another one, he was a sociable and talkative man, he used to talk to me nice" (Coser 1962, 59).

Nurses seem to perform a similar function. Patients rarely tend to mention the more technical aspects of nursing in describing a "good nurse."

. . . a good nurse "takes a personal interest in patients"; she should "help people all she can"; she should be "understanding and listen, not be impersonal"; she should "give attention to the patient" (Coser 1962, 70–71).

The most common complementary transactions between different levels are those that take place between parent and child. Playing the role of patient can reverse the traditional transaction between the biological parent and child.

> An elderly lady (in street clothes) is sitting at a table in the waiting room, eating her lunch. A younger lady (her daughter) sits next to her in an easy chair. Mother hands a portion of melon to daughter.
>
> *Daughter:* No, I won't eat it, you eat it.
>
> *Mother:* Please dearie, I can't.
>
> *Daughter:* Now you be a good girl and eat it. It's good for you.
>
> But mother still refuses and so daughter shrugs and humors her by taking a bite or two. Nurse's aide appears.
>
> *Daughter:* Go on, mother. You let the nurse take care of you. I'll wait here for you and see you later. You go now; I'll wait for you (Coser 1962, 41).

Such a transition is not always smooth. As indicated by the protest poem "Lament for My Lost Will" By Marie Woollcott (1961), the elderly, infirm relative can be as much of a headache for a family as the rebellious teenager.

Lament for My Lost Will

> I thought at twenty-one that freedom had begun:
> I was wrong.
> I am seventy-and-three and I'm very far from free;
> I would sell my so-called freedom for a song.
> I am slated, slated, slated
> To be daughter-dominated
> 'Til my will is constipated to the last degree.
> And it's long, long, long
> Since I've held my own opinion
> Or could sway my own dominion
> I am always overcome by the strong.
> Oh I know they love me dearly,
> And I know they wish me well,
> But I find I'm muttering queerly,
> "Go to Hell."
> If I want to pay the price
> I want to take my chance on vice
> When I choose to throw the dice.

I want to drink what I want to drink;
I want to think what I want to think;
I want to do what I want to do.
I WANT MY OWN POINT OF VIEW.

The most frequent parent-child game in health settings can be called *seed sowing*. This game involves a carefully concealed attempt to influence the behavior of an individual with higher status by feigning ignorance of what that person should do. More direct attempts to influence the behavior of a higher status person may be met by an icy rebuff such as, "Mr. Gonzales, *I'm* the administrator of this hospital," or, in the case of a nurse's attempts to influence, "Miss Jones, *I'm* the physician in charge of this patient." Individuals who meet with such responses know they have overstepped their bounds.

Seed sowing is an intricate game that requires a great deal of skill on the part of both parties if it is to be played effectively. However, if the players are skillful, the higher status physician or administrator will get the information he needs or will learn what to do in a particular situation without ever having to admit ignorance. At the same time the lower status person not only will obtain what he wants, but he may also derive a secret sense of superiority without the risk of direct conflict. Consider as examples the following opening lines of typical seed-sowing games.

Laundry supervisor: I really don't know what to do. We keep getting surgical instruments and bed pans dumped down the laundry chutes. It's dangerous, and we just don't know how to handle it.

Administrator: Hmm, I see you have a real problem. Let me see if I can figure out a way to handle it.

(The supervisor knows exactly what needs to be done, since he's talked with laundry supervisors in other hospitals. In the ensuing conversation, he will indirectly feed the solution to the administrator, who, if reasonably skillful, will pick it up and prescribe it as the appropriate course of action.)

Nurse: Doctor, I don't really know what to do with the patient in 304. We've tried everything from changing his diet to enemas.

Physician: Well, let's see, maybe I can write a prescription.

(The nurse hopes the physician will provide a laxative.)

Physician: Well, how are you feeling today?

Patient: I'm really feeling kind of irritable and out of sorts. Being in traction is kind of getting to me.

(The patient hopes the physician will eventually get the message and prescribe beer from the hospital pharmacy.)

The seed-sowing game becomes much more serious when a person's life is one of the stakes. Consider the following game between a green intern and a nurse faced with a patient with severe postpartum bleeding.

> . . . this woman was bleeding, I mean she was really gushing. She was just blanched out; her lips looked about the same color as her cheeks. She was conscious, but her pulse was fast and I couldn't even get a blood pressure reading, and she was panting for air and trying to sit up in bed, half-confused and picking at the bed sheets the way I had seen a couple of people do at Johns Hopkins when they were dying and knew it. . . . I stood there and thought, My God, she's just going to exsanguinate with me standing here holding her hand.
>
> Then one of the night nurses, bless her soul, said, "Doctor, I brought the shock blocks (wooden blocks used to elevate the foot of the bed to help combat shock) down here in case you might want them," and suddenly it dawned on me that it wasn't the bleeding I had to worry about right then, that this woman was in *shock*, and I said, "Yes, let's get those blocks under the foot of the bed." So two nurses shoved the shock blocks under the end of the bed while I lifted it up, tipping the woman's feet up at about a 30-degree angle. Then I started massaging her belly, trying to get the uterus to clamp down a little bit, and sent a nurse out to get an IV setup, and started trying to remember what you do for shock instead of what you do for postpartum hemorrhage. By now I was scared silly, and mad at myself as well; for all the dozens of times I had read about shock and what to do about it, I had never actually *seen* or *treated* a patient in shock, and at the moment I couldn't think of a damned thing.
>
> Then in a minute or two the nurse turned up with 1,000 cc's of 5 percent glucose water in an IV jug and said, "Doctor, if you're going to want to order any blood for this lady, maybe you can draw the blood sample for typing and cross-matching before you start the IV going," and again this gal saved the day—I hadn't even thought of a transfusion. I said, "Yes, I'm going to want three units of blood on an emergency cross-match," and then proceeded to draw the blood sample

for the blood bank to use for typing and cross-match and started the IV going. I knew about plasma expanders like dextran, but I was a little scared of them, and the woman was looking a little better now that her feet were tilted up, so I told the nurse to put some Pitocin in the IV, and when she said, "How much do you want in there?" I said, "Well, hell, enough to clamp that uterus down," and went back to the nurses' station with her. She told me they usually put an ampule of Pitocin in 1,000 cc's of glucose, so I said, "Fine, go ahead and do that," even though I didn't have the vaguest idea of how much Pitocin there was in an ampule (Doctor X 1965, 30–32).

Seed sowing can be facilitated by dispersing ideas among higher status individuals. Once the tacit support of one high-status person is obtained, the sower can be more direct in approaching other high-status persons. Citing the support of one high-status person provides great leverage for influencing others. Some hospital pharmacists are particularly adept at playing this game, widely sowing seeds among influential physicians, nursing staff, and administrators. With periodic contact and further fertilization, they are able to get their ideas adopted.

Crossed Transactions

While complementary transactions can be sustained indefinitely, as can the games that are built upon them, crossed transactions cannot. The two parties involved in a crossed transaction operate with very different expectations of one another. Two typical crossed transaction games are illustrated in figure 5.3. In order to sustain such transactions, the expectations involved must be transformed into complementary ones. Thus the game becomes one of seeing who will revert first to the other's expectations. This can be illustrated by looking at some opening moves in crossed transaction games.

Temper Tantrum

Admission clerk (adult to adult): I'm sorry, there aren't any beds available.
Physician, screaming over the telephone (child to parent): What the hell do you mean? I need a bed for this patient right now!

Clearly this transaction cannot be sustained. Either the physician or the admission clerk will have to alter his position. The admission

Figure 5.3   Typical Crossed Transaction Games

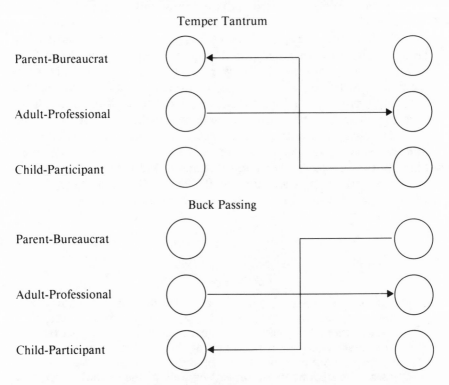

Temper Tantrum

Parent-Bureaucrat

Adult-Professional

Child-Participant

Buck Passing

Parent-Bureaucrat

Adult-Professional

Child-Participant

Adapted from: Berne, Eric. 1964. *Games People Play.* New York: Random House, p. 31.
Copyright © 1964. Reprinted by permission.

clerk can revert to a parent-child form of transaction and either attempt to placate the screaming child or retreat into bureaucratic-parental rigidity. The physician can revert to an adult-adult form of transaction and work with the clerk in a more objective, problem-solving manner. Another alternative would be for the clerk to become a child and revert to a temper tantrum himself, thereby forming a coalition with the physician against the institution. In any event, it is likely that a third party will have to be called in to resolve the confict.

Buck Passing

Patient (adult to adult): Look, I'd like to know what the diagnosis is.

Nurse (parent to child): You'll have to wait and talk to the doctor. I'm not supposed to discuss those things with you.

Buck-passing games pervade most large organizations, particularly health institutions, where responsibilities are unclear, knowledge fragmented, and prerogatives jealously guarded. In the exchange between the patient and nurse, the nurse could revert to an adult-adult pattern and simply provide the information the patient seeks. More likely, however, the nurse will attempt to impose a parent-child transaction on the situation, giving supportive reassurance to the patient but no information. In response, the patient will revert back to his position as a child. Many nurses, physicians, and administrators find it easier to withdraw and not engage in any transaction at all. The likelihood that such games will be engaged in is directly related to the seriousness of the diagnosis. Consequently, the cancer patient is one of the likeliest participants in such a game.

Institutionalized Practices
of Information Control

Nurses are remarkably adept at blocking patient inquiry about delicate matters by both verbal and nonverbal means, and an efficient professional demeanor checks many patients. Nurses are also successful much of the time in maintaining control of conversation in one of three ways: either they focus on the treatment and on getting well, or they avoid direct questions, or they talk about matters far removed from the hospital or the office. In the first instance, they use an occupationally determined strategy; in the others, they employ conversational devices brought from middle-class society in general. This professional rationale also serves an important self-protective function since the nurse can legitimately avoid seeking out information which is not essential for successful performance of her job and which, in fact, might make the job more difficult to accomplish were she better informed.

The physician's problem in face-to-face interaction is not so much how to avoid the topic altogether as it is how to give the patient sufficient information to insure cooperation in treatment and at the same time avoid unnecessary and prolonged scenes.

The use of evasion by physicians is directly related to a negative prognosis, but even those who more openly give concrete information to cancer patients are prone to use evasion in a subtle way. For example, the use of statistical chance to project a patient's future to the patient is an equivocation if family members are given a different account of the situation. The practice of giving incomplete and sometimes misleading information is supported by medical rationales which assert that the physician cannot deny hope to the patient, and the doctor who accepts this viewpoint can use various strategies to control the face-to-face interaction with his patients. For instance, he can focus complete attention on recovery, provide nonspecific answers to medical questions, avoid use of the word "cancer" and other potentially dangerous phrases, limit the time available for consultation, and refrain from discussing questions about the future. In addition, he can use his position to cut short conversation which threatens to become distressing or difficult to manage (Quint 1972, 232–33).

Games and Organizational Politics

Most games in organizational settings involve more than two parties. There are shifting coalitions designed to achieve certain goals or simply to provide personal protection. In this context, the games become political tactics that can be used to protect or further an individual's interests. The framework used to analyze two-party transactions is also useful in understanding these political tactics. Some of the more common tactics or games are described below. Just as with the two-party games, these tactics represent attempts by individuals to cope with organizations by protecting themselves and by attempting to control what happens within their organizations.

Godfather. This is a parent-child coalition in which the personal loyalty and small favors of the child are exchanged for protection and support. Such coalitions pervade all professional occupational groups. Old school and ethnic ties often help to cement such relationships. For example, a young physician might be assisted in getting a desirable internship, setting up his practice, or receiving certain hospital privileges by an older, influential physician-godfather.

[Dr. G] is an outstanding physician and heads the department of medicine in the big hospital. . . .

"When a person gets up to a position like mine there are a lot of kinds of help you can give your staff. I can always give a good fellow a couple of kicks in the right direction, I can always get an internship for a good boy if I really want to. I did that for M. I met him at a medical banquet while he was a student. I found out that he was a local boy and wanted an internship here. He was a nice sort with a good character. Now I've got him on the staff, and in a year or two I'm going to bring him into this office to share my practice. Then there was young Y. He was a nephew of the mayor. I got him an internship and the position of resident physician. . . ."

It is worth remarking that sponsorship has very few of the characteristics of nepotism. The protégé must live up to the expectations of his sponsor, he must "deliver the goods." Failure on his part would be more than personal failure—it would involve the prestige of his sponsor. The protégé is bound to go through the institutional apprenticeship. He must necessarily accept the discipline of being a functionary in an institution. Progressively he must accept the responsibilities of leadership. Sponsorship is by no means a one-sided set of favors (Hall 1948, 327–36).

Personal loyalties and family ties often result in such coalitions in the unskilled departments of hospitals as well. Unskilled employees who recruit relatives and friends to job openings are also playing godfather. In addition, godfathers' operations are not bounded by occupational group. For example, an influential physician might intercede on behalf of a hospital employee, cutting through the normal lines of authority.

Cover Your ———. Consultation and committee decision making are designed to help people arrive at optimal solutions to problems; they can also provide both emotional support and protection from the adverse consequences of a decision. In a sense, consultation and committee decision making represent a coalition of children against a potentially punitive parent. More cautious supervisors and administrators often adopt this as a managerial style. Physicians, too, have learned to adopt such procedures to protect themselves against rising malpractice suits.

The Doctor's New Dilemma—
Will I Be Sued?

"When an old patient told me that X-rays ordered by another doctor showed a cancer of the intestine, my first thought wasn't 'How will we treat it?' or 'I'm sorry to hear that,' but 'I'm sure I did a proctoscopy—but if I didn't, will I get sued?' I rushed back and checked my records, and I had done one just a month before, and felt completely O.K. I wouldn't be sued, I had done what was medically indicated and given the patient proper advice. It was a day or so before I realized that in my relief about not being vulnerable to suit I hadn't wondered about why I hadn't seen the tumor when I 'scoped her and that I still hadn't thought about therapy. I was ashamed of myself, but lawsuit—that's the first thing that leaps into your mind. . . ."

More expensive than the increasingly detailed consent forms are lab work, X-rays and hospitalization designed to prevent suits. At a recent pediatric meeting, Drs. Charles Shopfner and Fred Roberts of Kansas City reported a study of skull X-rays on children who appeared at their hospital complaining of head injuries. They concluded that the films have little diagnostic value, are wasteful of time and manpower and are taken primarily to protect the physician and hospital from lawsuits. Most doctors who work in emergency rooms are aware of the waste of time and resources involved in such films, but it is a very brave doctor indeed who dismisses without an X-ray a kid who fell out of a crib. Though the X-ray, whether positive or negative, probably will not affect treatment at all, if something goes wrong the doctor is going to look pretty weak on the witness stand without one. So the X-rays continue; juries are not miserly with crippled children. The emergency room's "proof" of a normal skull X-ray is at least some kind of defense, a demonstration that it followed standard procedures . . . (Halberstam 1971, 8, 35, 36).

While such defensive behavior sometimes provides patients greater protection, it is costly and often inconclusive. At worst, this tactic can cause individuals to invest more and more energy in protecting themselves and less and less in what they are actually responsible for doing, a situation that can lead eventually to paralysis within an institution.

Blame the Victim. In a sense, blame the victim is the opposite of cover your —— because it represents a coalition of parents against a child. In this game, rather than accept a shared responsibility for foul-ups, a group of people will place the blame on the lowest status person involved. For example, a patient's failure to keep clinic appointments or to follow prescribed treatment is likely to be blamed on the patient.

It is unfortunate that much of the research on patient behavior has reinforced the tendency of providers to blame the patient for ineffective utilization of care. A great deal of research has been done on the psychological and cultural differences between effective and ineffective users. Ineffective users tend to be lower class persons or members of ethnic minorities, or both, and these people often face a very different system of care. Supportive services such as medical social work, rehabilitation, and mental health programs help assure the most effective use of health care services, and yet such programs are far less likely to exist in hospitals in poorer communities than in hospitals in wealthier areas (Smith and Kaluzny 1974).

Another frequent victim in health care organizations is the unskilled or semiskilled worker, who is delegated limited technical tasks but is assumed by more professionally skilled staff members to have broader responsibilities. Inadequate explanations and controls are often the true culprits responsible for foul-ups in these situations.

Smoke Bomb. This tactic involves trying to avoid adult-adult transactions by replacing them with parent-child transactions. This is achieved by emphasizing the complexities of a particular situation, throwing up a lot of technical jargon, and presenting as many real or imagined technical arguments in opposition to a proposed action as possible. Many planning agency staff studies of bed and facility needs fall victim to this tactic. It is relatively easy for providers to poke technical holes in such studies, since the state of the art limits the precision of them and their recommendations. Too often the actions of providers remain unaffected by such research efforts because of "methodological" problems.

Quality review programs that threaten to impinge on the prerogatives of individual physicians are also assaulted. For example, the inadequacy of various methods of record review and the inappropriateness of statistical analysis are attacked; instead, emphasis is placed on the idea that medicine is an art that cannot be subjected to quantification without gross distortion. The Peer Review Organization (PRO), which provides for monitoring of medical practice, has been attacked on this basis by spokesmen for organized medicine and hospitals.

A similar tactic is often used by administrators in their battles against unionization of nonprofessional employees. In these transactions, paternalistic appeals are combined with descriptions of the serious problems that could result from unionization.

Co-optation. This is a classic tactic used by bureaucracies to deal with participants (children). It involves transforming children into professionals or bureaucrats by assigning them appropriate tasks and granting them all the trimmings that go along with such tasks. The creation of new committees and community advisory groups are examples of this tactic. Eventually the co-opted persons begin to acquire the values and orientations of the professionals and bureaucrats with whom they were once in conflict.

End Run. The end run is probably the most dangerous tactic in which an individual can engage. It involves a coalition of children against parents that extends beyond the boundaries of the institution. Those engaged in this tactic violate both professional and bureaucratic norms, and unless they are very successful in building their coalition or in concealing their identities, they are likely to be fired. However, there are less dangerous forms of the end run (such as selectively leaking information to the press or to outside groups), and these are part of the day-to-day life in most organizations.

SUMMARY AND CONCLUSIONS

The games that individuals play are similar to the search procedures of organizations. When an individual is faced with a conflict between his own needs and goals and those of an organization he is part of, the individual will first (1) attempt to alter or manipulate the environment (for example, attempt to gain sympathy from the supervisor for being late), then (2) make minimal adjustments (show up on time for work), and finally either (3) make basic changes in his own goals and remain within the organization or (4) leave for a more compatible position or unemployment. The degree of difficulty and the resulting degree of stress rise geometrically as one progresses from stage 1 to stage 4. Individual change, like organizational change, means giving up what is comfortable and possibly losing control.

Under such circumstances, resistance is rational. Stress arises when an individual (or organization) is called upon to respond to a situation with some sort of coping behavior but he is either unable or uncertain that he will be able to do so. The subsequent psychological and physical arousal, the "fight or flight" response, triggers biochemical (organizational) changes that are instrumental in causing a variety of pathologies, including most of the major causes of death—coronary heart disease, stroke, and cancer. The connections between stress, hypertension, and ulcers and between drugs, alcohol, and accidental deaths are well documented (Terris 1976).

Organizations experience similar stress when required to adapt to change. In the case of organizations, the pathologies include high rates of turnover and absenteeism as well as other problems with employee morale. It also involves an increase in the kind of errors that can adversely affect the organization's ability to survive. The critical issue is how to balance individual and organizational needs against demands for rapid change. We will discuss that in the next chapter.

6

Accommodation

Vanity and careful training
Blind those to the maiming
Who have learned the question
Only the lunch for indigestion.

Power can either hold organizations and social systems together or tear them apart. It is most visible in the negotiations that assure the organization gets what it needs from its members in exchange for meeting their needs. The health system represents a complex network of such exchanges. For example, a nurse may have a contract with a hospital to receive a salary in return for work performed during a particular shift on a particular floor of the hospital. The hospital, in turn, may have a contract with a health insurance company for payment of part of the costs of employing this nurse in return for providing hospital care for the health insurance plan's subscribers. The health insurance plan may have a contract with a company to provide such hospital benefits to its employees. This, in turn, may result from a collective bargaining agreement negotiated between the company and the union representing the employees. The power of each of these parties is reflected in the strength of its bargaining position in such negotiations.

In chapter 4 we described the particular orientation and concerns that an organization brings to such negotiations with the major elements of its environment. In chapter 5 we described the particular orientations that individuals bring to negotiations of their roles within an organization. In this final chapter on organizational structure, we will describe the sources of power available to each of the participants in such negotiations and the accommodations that result.

Figure 6.1 Flow of Power in the Health Care System

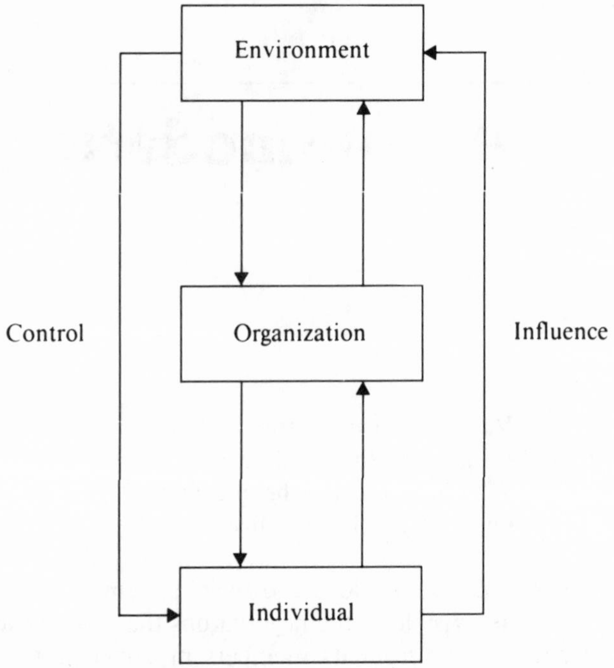

```
                    ┌─────────────────────┐
              ┌─────┤     Environment      │◄────┐
              │     └─────────┬────────────┘     │
              │               │              ▲   │
              │               │              │   │
              │               ▼              │   │
              │     ┌─────────────────────┐  │   │
  Control     │     │    Organization     │  │   │   Influence
              │     └─────────┬───────────┘  │   │
              │               │              ▲  │
              │               │              │  │
              │               ▼              │  │
              │     ┌─────────────────────┐  │  │
              └────►│     Individual       ├──┘  │
                    └─────────────────────┘
```

ORGANIZATIONAL CONTRACTS

The conflicting demands of the environment, the organization, and the individual are diagramed in figure 6.1. In order for them to satisfy their needs, they must arrive at some form of accommodation with each other. That accommodation, or contract, may be an informal agreement or an explicit legal document that spells out the respective rights and obligations of each party. The arrows in figure 6.1 represent power, or the ability of a party to obtain through such negotiations and exchanges something it would not have obtained otherwise. On the one hand, such power can be exerted by the organization to hold things together and make them work—that is, to achieve, in the traditional managerial sense, *control* (the arrows pointing downward). On the other hand, such power can also be exercised by individuals or smaller organizations without any regard for the impact on larger structures. Thus who gets what when, where, and how, or *influence* (the arrows pointing upward), is the traditional political science perspective on power.

Organizations and systems can survive only by balancing these opposing forces (Gamson 1968, Hirschman 1970). Organizations that offer no advantage over the same activities performed by an individual will cease to exist. Physicians, for example, tend to join groups rather than to practice solo when such arrangements provide greater efficiency in marketing their services. The "brand name" of a recognized specialty group is particularly useful, since the public has little information on which to base judgments of relative quality. Hence, the preponderance of medical groups is specialty-based, whereas most solo practice is done by general practitioners (Getzen 1981).

The same self-interest that creates organizations tends to undermine them. Individual opportunism erodes the efficiency of cooperative behavior. Effective control becomes more difficult, and attempts to exert it may result in the disintegration of the organization. HMOs, for example, which depend on the support and cooperation of their medical staffs for the competitive position and growth necessary for their survival, have experienced difficulty, even when their development was subsidized by federal grants. For example, 37 out of 79 HMOs that were awarded development grants between 1971 and 1973 and 49 of 108 that were awarded feasibility grants in 1975 were disbanded (Stumpf 1976). Disagreements over income distribution among physicians played a major role in many of these dissolutions. Either the expected financial gains did not materialize or there was squabbling over the profits. On the other hand, physician groups that are formed primarily out of concern for providing better service and developing higher professional standards seem to result in more stable organizations (Dubois 1967).

All organizations experience centrifugal forces, and there are two ways they can combat them (Ouchi 1977). First, they can foster a sense of trust and a sense of mutual support among the members. The goals are to have no member feel that the others are cynically exploiting his efforts and to have all members feel that everyone shares in the benefits of cooperative activity. This is the strategy adopted by participatory and, to a lesser extent, professional organizations. Among medical groups, giving members greater influence in decisions related to practice and placing greater emphasis on the quality of the services provided appear to assure greater stability (Dubois 1967).

Second, organizations can assume that members are incapable of any behavior other than opportunism. They can develop close monitoring, punishment, and greater specialization to keep such behavior within acceptable bounds. This is the philosophy underlying the control structure of bureaucratic organizations. Physicians in a group, for example, could be forced to punch time clocks and meet strict productivity standards (measured in number of patient visits per hour). Such procedures are far easier to create than a climate of trust. They are also far more in keeping with the cultural environment in which most organizations operate.

There are two disadvantages of such an approach. First, employees can leave the organization. The ease with which they can do this depends on the market for their skills and their geographic mobility. Since physicians can leave relatively easily, this approach is rarely tried. Nursing shortages have stalled similar efforts at control of nursing departments in some regions of the country. Second, rigid controls exact a heavy price from the individuals subjected to them. They heighten stress because of the job insecurity they produce. Further, the division of labor tends to eliminate much of the enjoyment individuals get from doing their work. The rapid pace of production adds to physical stress and reduces the opportunity for pleasurable social interaction with co-workers. All of these factors increase the stress individuals experience at work, and, since the most common causes of disability and death appear to be related to stress, seem likely to increase the rates of death and disability among employees (Eyer 1977). This may, in turn, reduce the productivity and effectiveness of an organization.

What makes rigid control cost-effective from the standpoint of the organization, however, is that the organization usually gets stuck with paying only a small part of the cost of such stress—just as in the past corporations did not have to pay the cost of polluting the air and water. Whether organizations whose reason for existence is to make people healthy should pursue such control strategies is a troublesome issue.

Organizations that adopt rigid control strategies will devise ways to avoid paying as much of the cost of such strategies as possible. Hospitals, for example, have collaborated both formally and informally in setting wage and work standards, particularly for nurses, to keep them from leaving. This strategy has not prevented nurses from leaving the profession altogether, however, thus creating periodic shortages of nurses. Although rarely articulated, comprehensive employer-paid health insurance benefits ensure that the employer pays at least part of the social cost of the way the organization exploits human resources. Not surprisingly, there is increasing pressure from local business coalitions to force greater copayments from employees and to restrict employers' payments even further.

Relative bargaining strength, or power, largely determines which strategy for controlling opportunism is adopted. In organizations where members tend to have a great deal of influence, efforts will be made to create a climate of trust. In an organization or segments of organizations in which individuals have relatively little influence, a more bureaucratic strategy for control will be adopted. In organizations where there are wide variations in the amount of power individuals or groups have (as in most health care settings), a contingency approach to organizational control is adopted. Physicians, for example, are controlled through more participatory means, whereas semiskilled service workers are subjected to the rigors of bureaucratic discipline. While these differences in control are often attributed to the nature of the work and the technology, they are also related to the relative power of the individuals and groups involved.

These two control strategies reflect two fundamentally different perceptions of power in organizations (Ng 1980, 60–73). Power can be perceived as a limited resource to be struggled for in a zero-sum game, or it can be perceived as a resource limited only by human imagination, one that can be expanded with use. In either case, power is a resource that individuals and societies lend to organizations to use for their benefit and, like a bank account, that they never relinquish ownership of. Most decisions and activities of organizations are routine and incremental and fit the second set of perceptions well. Conflict-related decisions are relatively rare (Hage 1980, 54–56), yet most managers and, indeed, most members of organizations see power as a zero-sum game. Bureaucratic models of organizations tend to reinforce this perception, whereas participatory and professional models tend to perceive power differently, recognizing the value of influence as well as control in enhancing overall power and effectiveness. These differences are illustrated in figure 6.2, which was originally used to classify different leadership styles and orientations in organizations (Blake and Mouton 1967).

If one assumes that the amount of power within an organization is fixed, then any greater degree of organizational control must be extracted from the influence of individual participants. Managerial concern for participants and for production are consequently in conflict. Organizational life consists of an ongoing struggle between the establishment of an organizational structure and managerial style that are responsive to the needs of individual participants (*1,9*) and a structure and style that allow the desires and needs of individuals to interfere least (*9,1*). Bureaucratic structures attempt to achieve control at the expense of the influence of individual participants.

If, on the other hand, one assumes that power in an organization is not fixed and limited, that it is expandable, then greater influence of participants and organizational control need not be incompatible. Given such an assumption, organizations can progress from structures

Figure 6.2   Distribution of Power Within Organizations and the Resulting Alternatives for Managerial Style, under Assumptions of Fixed and Expandable Power

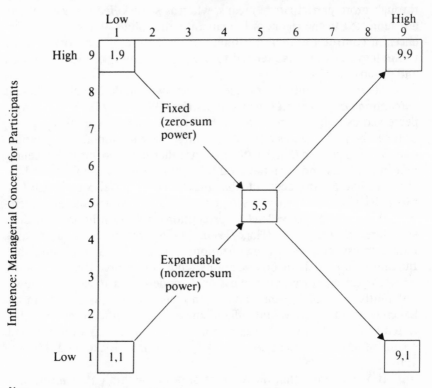

Control: Managerial Concern for Production

Key

1.1: Exertion of the minimum effort to get the required work done is sufficient to sustain membership in the organization.

1.9: Thoughtful attention to participants' needs for satisfying relationships leads to comfortable, friendly organizational atmosphere and work tempo.

5.5: Adequate organizational performance is possible by balancing the necessity of getting work done and of maintaining satisfactory morale.

9.1: Efficiency results from arranging the conditions of work in such a way that the human element interferes minimally.

9.9: Interdependent, committed participants have a common stake in the organization's goals, leading to relationships of trust and respect.

Adapted from: Blake and Mouton 1967, 12–47. Reprinted by permission.

and managerial styles that are neither particularly responsive to the needs of individual participants nor particularly efficient (*1,1*) toward structures and styles that are very responsive and efficient (*9,9*). Participatory and, to a lesser extent, professional structures tend to operate under this assumption. They tend to recognize the reciprocal nature of the exchange between individuals and organizations that bureaucratic structures ignore. In the next section we explain how power is acquired and used.

SOURCES OF POWER

Power in any negotiating situation is determined by dependency. The more dependent A is on what B can provide and the less dependent B is on what A can provide, the more powerful B is. We will show how this works for the individual, the organization, and the organization's environment.

Individual Power

Individuals are able to limit the power organizations have over them by limiting their dependency on the organizations. Individuals who can leave an organization easily, as in the case of physicians and nurses, force greater accommodation from the organization. At the same time, individuals acquire power within organizations by enhancing the organization's dependence on them through their (1) expert knowledge, (2) position within the organization, and (3) absorption of residual tasks that are important for the effective functioning of the organization.

Expert Power. Persons with skills that are essential to the functioning of an organization possess power, regardless of their formal positions within the hierarchy. This power can be protected by developing a professional structure that controls access to these skills or knowledge. The claim to a unique body of knowledge makes it impossible for outsiders to pass judgment on professional performance. It is professional control, this claim to a specialized body of knowledge, that has enabled physicians to maintain their considerable autonomy.

Physicians are not the only persons who wield expert power in health care settings, nor is expert power limited to persons with "professional" credentials, as the experience of one self-trained electronics wizard suggests.

A large teaching hospital was faced with an increasing problem as a result of its growing dependence on complex electronic equipment on the nursing floors. Frequent malfunctions would disrupt the floor routines. The nursing staff were not sufficiently knowledgeable to repair the equipment, and often the maintenance people were equally inept. One day a small, wiry, intense nineteen-year-old boy with thick steel-rimmed glasses and long straggly hair arrived on the scene. In true Walter Mitty fashion he breezed from floor to floor fixing almost instantaneously all kinds of failing equipment with little more than a pen knife. His reputation spread throughout the hospital, and he was treated with a certain awe by the nurses and other maintenance employees, for whom he was quite adept at expressing his contempt. Olsen, his supervisor, a former construction foreman complete with cigar, tattoos, American flag decal on his windshield, and a tough, machismo supervisory style, found his new charge a difficult pill to swallow. Things soon came to a head, and Olsen stormed into the director's office screaming: "Either that damn punk kid gets the axe or you can shove this whole hospital up your ———! It's either him or me!"

A meeting was then called with the administrative staff, the boy wizard, and Olsen to figure out a way of working out their differences. Olsen soon lost his temper, labeling the proceedings "bullshit," among other things. When Olsen paused to catch his breath, the boy wizard rose and said calmly, "I was expecting this." He then pulled out a can of air freshener spray relabeled "bullshit spray," squirted Olsen in the face with it, announced his immediate resignation, and, with impeccable dignity, marched out of the room.

The next morning the director found a group of nurses sitting in his office demanding the reinstatement of the wizard.

The wizard was rehired at a considerably higher salary the following day and was placed in a different department, where he was essentially insulated from any direct supervision. A half-hearted effort was made to obscure these maneuvers in such a way that Olsen would not lose face. Such is the power of the expert.

Positional Power. Persons in positions of responsibility in a bureaucracy are given authority (legitimized power) to carry out the control activities necessary to meet those responsibilities. Other individuals in the organization and the organization itself thus depend on such persons to accomplish organizational objectives. This is the only power that is officially recognized in bureaucratic institutions. Depending on the degree of professionalism in the organization, however, formal positions may have little actual power. Relatively weak individuals, persons with little personal influence over subordinates, can perform routine functions adequately without getting in the hair of professionals. Indeed, by awarding supervisory positions on the basis of seniority or other qualities not likely to disrupt the routines of professionals, the more ambitious, domineering individuals are screened out.

As organizations grow in size and complexity and as the emphasis on cost control increases, positional power assumes far greater importance in program and budgeting decisions. The position itself begins to confer expert status because it requires an ability to negotiate projects and solve problems within an increasingly complex organizational system (Mintzberg 1979).

Residual Power. Residual power, that which is not assumed by professionals or by position in the hierarchy, is up for grabs. It can be acquired by controlling access to (1) information, (2) key individuals within the organization, or (3) the physical plant or essential equipment (Mechanic 1962). Such power is often possessed by persons in relatively routine, unskilled, low-status positions. For example, the admissions clerk in the outpatient department wields a great deal of power over those patients, since he or she alone regulates access to physicians. Secretaries of administrators and department heads wield similar power over accessibility, as well as having access to information that many persons in higher positions lack.

Residual power is enhanced when individuals develop special knowledge about the organization that higher-ups have little interest in acquiring and when they are perceived as trustworthy by these same higher-ups, who then delegate increased responsibility to them. Their power is enhanced even further if they are physically close to key sources of information or resources. The secretary of an administrator, for example, can, within limits, control access to the boss, as well as the distribution of information to subordinates. Over time, more discretion will tend to be given such a secretary, and she or he will absorb more power. In cases where the boss is inept or disinterested, the secretary can end up as de facto head of the institution.

Health services organizations generally provide ample opportunity for acquiring residual power, because decisions tend to be made by committees and because many health professionals cannot tolerate administrative detail and routines. The pattern of decision making in such professionally dominated organizations follows what some observers have described as the garbage can model. In this model, a random stream of decision makers merges with a random stream of problems and a random stream of solutions to produce a random stream of decisions, or pairings of problems with solutions (Cohen, March, and Olsen 1972). This process allows individuals who are willing to help shape the randomness of these respective streams to acquire residual power. In many settings, the process has enabled administrators to exercise a good deal of influence over an institution's medical staff. Such power can also be exercised by individuals at the bottom of the organization, as illustrated in the following description of how attendants in a psychiatric ward consistently subverted efforts at reform.

Ward Attendant Control in a Mental Hospital

Repeated efforts to transform the custodial character of a 4,000-bed 100-year-old state psychiatric institution into a "therapeutic community" foundered. The radical reforms had the full support of both the hospital's administration and its medical staff. Yet each new initiative was effectively blocked by the low-paid, relatively untrained, and presumably powerless ward attendants. How was this possible?

The key to control of the ward attendants was the ward physician, the only representative of the administration on most wards. There was high turnover among ward physicians, and, through administrative policy, they were reassigned to different wards as many as five times a year. In contrast, ward attendants had a long tenure and little turnover in their positions. In addition, the ward physicians were woefully unprepared for such a responsibility and viewed any time spent outside of individual psychotherapy or medical treatment as an irritating distraction from their "real job."

Since the physicians had other demands on their time besides floor supervision, they were dependent on the attendants to carry out the day-to-day activities on the floor. The ward attendants were consequently able to make the ward physician their captive or force him to quit. If displeased with the efforts of the physician to alter the environment on the floor, the ward attendants could withhold from him information that he needed to assess the patients. The ward attendants could also manipulate the flow of patients requesting the attention of the physician, creating near–mob scenes and making it difficult for the physician to leave the ward. Most important, they could withhold their cooperation in the treatment of the 150 patients the ward physician was legally responsible for. Simply changing dosage of tranquilizers would absorb a good proportion of the physician's time.

The physician would either knuckle under or find his position intolerable and quit. In turn, the administration was forced to relax its pressure on physicians to implement the reforms. As a result, the ward staff, with neither positional or expert power, remained firmly in control of what happened in the institution (Sheff 1961, 93–105; paraphrased).

Group Power

This isn't really an organization, it's a city. There are different factions and political parties pursuing their own special interests, each relating to a different constituency—many of which are outside the hospital—and all tugging in different directions. I feel sorry for anybody who tries to put it together and make sense out of it.

Maintenance man in a large teaching hospital

Much of the actual power that exists within an organization, as suggested by the description of the ward attendants in the psychiatric hospital, is generated from the mosaic of groups that make up the organization. Most are invisible on an organizational chart yet essential to efficient operation. These groups present the most difficult problems in holding an organization together. A "group" is any number of people who interact with each other and who perceive themselves as members of a group (Schein 1972). Groups share common work, interests, or goals. Interest groups or coalitions cut across organizational boundaries and at times pursue goals that are inconsistent with those of the organization. For example, the "groupiness" of some board members and medical staff who belong to the same social clubs often enables them to circumvent the hospital hierarchy. The radiologists on staff at a hospital might band together and operate a private laboratory in their off hours that would eventually compete directly with the hospital's laboratory. On the other hand, bringing departmental supervisors together and making them feel that they are part of a problem-solving group can do much to reduce problems of coordination between departments that would be slow and cumbersome to deal with more formally. Judicious promotions and appointments to key committees often help administrators shape the development and direction of coalitions (Pfeffer 1981).

All groups exert a great deal of influence over their members. They satisfy needs that could not be satisfied by the formal organization and, consequently, can create strong loyalties. They fill needs for friendship and support, provide a way of confirming one's sense of identity and self-esteem, supply a safe way of defining and testing organizational realities, help increase an individual's sense of security and power, and may even help make the actual tasks required easier.

> Hospital laundry workers have always had perhaps the dirtiest, most unpleasant job in a hospital. The laundry, usually located in a hot, poorly ventilated corner of the hospital's subbasement, provides a small, physically cramped work space. In the summer the heat may become unbearable. The task of removing laundry—often soaked in blood or reeking of urine, feces, or vomit—from the laundry chutes and placing it in the washing machines is often complicated by having to remove the soiled scalpels, bedpans, and so on that are inadvertently dumped down the chutes.

> The employees in housekeeping would seem to have a better deal. The pay is comparable to that of laundry workers, and the work itself is usually lighter and carried out in more pleasant physical surroundings. Yet turnover and absenteeism, often a constant headache in urban hospitals, is much higher among housekeeping personnel than among laundry workers. Individuals hired as laundry workers seem to stay, often spending much of their working life in this environment. Why? What is it about the laundry that fosters group rewards not available to housekeeping personnel?

Strong group loyalty can solve the problems of absenteeism and turnover, but it can be a two-edged sword. A tightly knit work group can also block the achievement of the larger goals of an organization. Look at what happened when the laundry workers felt threatened.

> The administration of a large teaching hospital concluded that substantial savings could be obtained in the long run by purchasing from a German manufacturer an automated laundry system. It was explained to the laundry workers that none of them would be laid off, although some might eventually be placed in other departments within the hospital through normal attrition in these areas. It was not clear, however, how much of this message got through, since most of the laundry workers were Puerto Rican and some had difficulty understanding English. These communication problems were not helped by the German mechanics who arrived and started to install the new automated unit. The mechanics had a great deal of difficulty getting things to work. Things

kept going wrong, things that could go wrong only with a little help from the laundry workers. The system's first year of operation was a disaster. For the first time laundry had to be shipped out to a commercial laundry, since parts of the system were always breaking down. There was no love lost between the laundry workers and the German mechanics by the end of that year.

In the end, however, the laundry workers lost. Too much power was marshalled against them. The system was finally made to work, and the remaining laundry workers were forced to accept it. For other groups, such a technological innovation in the name of efficiency might never have been attempted. The power of a work group to control its own activities (assuming that, unlike the case of the ward attendants, no residual power exists) depends on how predictable and well understood the tasks it performs are. That predictability left the laundry workers with little power to define and organize their own work. On the other hand, if the tasks performed by a group are nonroutine and not well understood by outsiders, the group will have a great deal more freedom in the way it defines and organizes work.

In general, those groups that perform the most critical tasks have the most influence. The characteristics and ideology of these groups are inevitably reflected in the policies and goals of the institution. The most critical tasks will shift from time to time (Perrow 1963). For example, until the 1930s, the most critical task for assuring the survival of most hospitals was to assure sufficient local contributions to enable them to continue their predominantly charitable mission. Nor surprisingly, trustees and boards of directors, the major conduit for such contributions, were dominant in hospital governance. With the development of insurance mechanisms and the rapid advancements in scientific medicine in the 1930s, local charitable contributions became a less critical resource, and the need to be at the forefront of scientific advances gained in importance. The medical staff, particularly members with strong academic reputations, became the dominant force within many hospitals.

Finally, from the 1950s on, issues of internal coordination and of access to capital and third-party payment of operating expenses have grown in importance; with this trend, administrators have grown in importance. A multiple leadership structure emerged in many facilities —one in which the board, the administrator, and the medical staff have relatively insulated spheres of influence. Such a structure makes long-range planning and decisions about resource allocation, which are likely to uncover conflicting interests, difficult to make. Given the new financial strains making it harder to provide "something for everyone" and the emergence of multi-institutional arrangements, this structure appears to be breaking down. What the outcome is likely to be is unclear. On the one hand, administrators have assumed corporate titles like president or chief executive officer, and many hospitals have been reorganized along the single line of authority that exists in private corporate structures. On the other hand, development of governing boards responsible for multiple institutions appears to limit the control of individual administrators (Alexander and Morlock 1985). Tenure in many of these new corporate positions has become far more precarious. In one recent year in Pennsylvania, for example, there was an almost 20 percent turnover of chief executive officers of hospitals. Most recent hospital association surveys of membership indicate that governance has become the most difficult and perplexing problem faced by administrators.

Organizational Power

> It is an astonishment, which every patient feels from time to time, observing the affairs of a large, complex hospital from the vantage point of his bed, that the whole institution doesn't fly to pieces. A hospital operates by a constant interplay of powerful forces essential to getting necessary things done, but always at odds with each other. The intern staff is an almost irresistible force in itself, learning medicine by doing medicine, assuming all the responsibility within reach, pushing against an immovable attending and administrative staff, and frequently at odds with the nurses. The attending physicians are individual entrepreneurs trying to run small cottage industries at each bedside. The diagnostic laboratories are feudal fiefdoms, prospering from the insatiable demands for their services from interns and residents. The medical students are all over the place, learning as best they can and complaining that they are not, as they believe they should be, at the epicenter of everyone's concern. Each individual worker in the place, from the chiefs of surgery to the dieticians to the ward maids, porters and elevator operators, lives and works in the conviction that the whole apparatus would come to a standstill without his or her individual contribution, and, in one sense or another, each of them is right (Thomas 1983, 66).

So far, we have talked about power from the perspective of the individual. We now look at power from the control side, or the ability of the organization to extract what it needs from the individuals and groups that work within it. Organizations work because effective control holds various individuals and groups together and makes it possible for larger organizational goals to be achieved. Whatever this glue is that holds health institutions together, it does not appear to work as well as it has in the past. We will review the possible sources of such power to control members of organizations and suggest some reasons for the apparent breakdown of control in the health sector.

The most difficult control problems an organization faces are usually related to controlling persons at the lowest levels of the organization. Although it is a somewhat simplistic scheme, organizations can be classified by type of power used to gain compliance from, or control over, such persons. This power may be predominantly coercive, remunerative, or normative (Etzioni 1961).

A *coercive* control mechanism is one that uses (or threatens to use) physical force to gain compliance from persons on the lower levels. Concentration camps, traditional prisons, and mental hospitals are the classic examples of such organizaitons. In the health care sector, as in society as a whole, such methods of control are required only for deviates, the violent mental patient requiring physical restraint or the employee involved in kickback schemes.

A *remunerative* control mechanism depends on allocation of material rewards such as wages, salaries, and bonuses to assure compliance. This is usually the major part of the contract that is negotiated between the individual and an organization. It is also central to most policy debates concerning how to control health care providers. It is assumed that all that is needed to assure correct behavior on the part of providers is correct financial incentive.

A *normative* control mechanism depends on shared values. In this case, the individual will accept the directives of the organization not because he fears physical punishment or desires financial gain, but because he has accepted and internalized the goals of the organization. Churches and many voluntary associations, including the traditional hospital as well as newly formed holistic health centers, tend to rely predominantly on such mechanisms of control. Some would argue that internalization of the values of the organization is the key factor in the Japanese approach to management (Ouchi 1981). Such organizations presumably combine the high degree of participant influence and organizational control of the *9,9* style of management described in figure 6.2.

To be most effective, an organization's ends (its goals) must be compatible with its means (control mechanisms). If maintaining order is the primary goal of an organization, then a coercive control structure will be most effective. Psychiatric facilities for the criminally insane that rely primarily on the shared beliefs and values of patients and officials to assure control of patients will probably be in trouble. If the goal of an organization is to produce goods for a profit, then utilitarian control structures will probably be most effective. Appeals for moral commitment or threats of punishment will probably not be effective in gaining compliance from physicians in solo fee-for-service practices. The appeals would be ignored, and the threats would not be tolerated. On the other hand, if the goals are cultural, normative control structures will probably be most effective. A professional association that attempted to attract and hold members either by threats of force or by financial incentives would not be very effective in achieving its goals.

It requires far more effort to create and maintain normative control structures than coercive or remunerative ones. In order to be effective, normative controls require a high degree of consensus and intense moral involvement from the members of an organization. All that is necessary for remunerative control structures to work is the calculated involvement of the lower-level participants in an organization and the ability of the organization to meet the participants' material needs. Coercive control structures require no positive involvement on the part of lower-level participants, who almost by definition are alienated from the goals of the organization.

In order to develop normative control structures, the organization must pay a great deal of attention to indoctrination and training. Such training tends to be lengthy and emphasizes the values of the organization as well as the technical skills required for a particular job. Such approaches have been adopted by many of the most successful private corporations and have been viewed by some as a key factor in their success (Peters and Waterman 1982). Purely remunerative organizations, on the other hand, tend to delegate training in technical skills to outside institutions, with little concern about inculcating organizational values. In coercive organizations, there is little need for either inculcating organizational values or teaching technical skills.

Effective leadership, predictably, is far more difficult to achieve within normative control structures. Leaders must not only make certain that the objective tasks of the organization are performed but also assure that the social cohesion of participants is maintained. Adequate communication is crucial to both. Most health care institutions today are racked with disputes and show an increasing lack of common purpose, other than a remunerative one, which tends to be divisive. Just as the medical groups that tended to focus on the remunerative aspects of their association deteriorated, so other health service organizations with that focus are being pulled apart. In spite of all the conflicting interests in a complex teaching hospital, it is shared values that hold it together. It is ironic that, while successful private corporations have discovered the importance of investing in normative aspects of control, health care organizations have attempted to become more "businesslike" and remunerative in their control structures.

System Power

Just as mutually advantageous "contracts" are negotiated between individuals and organizations, so contracts bind organizations that provide health services to organizations that shape their environment. It is through interorganizational contracts that the power relationships and structure of the overall system are defined. Most third-party payers and providers of care, for example, enter into precise legal contracts that spell out their respective rights and obligations. For the hospital, these contracts provide a predictable stream of patients and funds that assure it of meeting its financial obligations. For the third-party insurance carrier, the contract provides a way for it to meet its obligations to enrollees. Just as an individual who is dissatisfied with his role in an organization can leave, so a provider organization that believes the contract is not satisfactory can choose not to participate. For example, physicians may choose not to accept Medicaid patients and, with Medicare, not to accept assignment (direct billing of Medicare by the physician and acceptance of the Medicare payment as payment in full). Hospitals and nursing homes can make similar decisions, although they seldom do, because they are far more dependent on Medicaid and Medicare care for their revenues than are physicians in private practice.

The lack of contracts between Blue Cross plans and local hospitals has caused difficulties. In some instances, negotiations have broken down completely, and no contract was signed. The hospitals attempted to collect what they believed were reasonable charges directly from patients, and patients, caught between Blue Cross and the hospital, had to pay out of pocket those charges that Blue Cross would not pay. The resulting dissatisfaction threatened Blue Cross contracts with major employers and, consequently, Blue Cross's market share. The hospitals faced cumbersome and serious collection problems they were not equipped to handle. Clearly, neither Blue Cross nor the hospitals can afford, at least in the short run, to fail to reach agreement.

In any contract negotiation process, each party attempts to improve its bargaining position. This is done, just as in negotiations between the individual and the organization, by reducing A's dependency on B while enhancing B's dependency on A. In the example of Blue

Cross contracts with hospitals, Blue Cross plans have entered into cost-containment coalitions with major businesses to assure that bargaining goes on in a cost-conscious environment and to tie the business community to the insurance carrier in such a way as to prevent the erosion of market share. At the same time, many Blue Cross plans have attempted to diversify by setting up other businesses, including operations that compete directly with hospitals on some fronts—namely, HMOs, home care programs, and so on. Hospitals have used a similar strategy in attempting to make themselves less dependent on Blue Cross. Recognizing that there is strength in numbers, many regional hospital associations bargain collectively for their members. In some states, they have also tacitly supported all-payer legislation, which erodes Blue Cross's market share by making commercial insurance plans more competitive in price and making the hospital less dependent on a single third-party source of payment. Some hospitals have helped sponsor prepayment plans that compete directly with Blue Cross, and others have entered into a variety of ventures that completely insulate them from inpatient payment mechanisms. For example, they may provide services to other providers, or they may develop ancillary services for discharged patients, such as rental of medical equipment or providing oxygen tanks for home use.

> One particularly lucrative area for hospital business expansion, designed to make it less dependent on inpatient revenues from third parties such as Blue Cross, has been the medical equipment rental market. Third parties, and particularly Medicare, have up until now focused on inpatient cost controls and have provided fairly comfortable ceilings in terms of payment. A crutch that costs $20, for example, can be rented to a discharged patient for $7 a month. Where else can the cost of a capital investment be recovered in less than three months? This may seem like a nickel-and-dime candy store operation, and many administrators have ignored it because of this. [Several of these freestanding for-profit nickel-and-dime candy store operators in Philadelphia sold their businesses last year and became multimillionaires.] On the average, a discharged hospital patient referred to one of these operations rents three to four different pieces of equipment (bed, respirator, and so on) in addition to consumables, such as oxygen, producing an average gross income per referral of as much as $1,000. These referrals have come often at the price of some Christmas candy for the social workers. Many hospitals are now getting a bigger piece of the action, setting up their own subsidiaries to provide these supplies to pa-

tients or entering into joint ventures with particular suppliers, from which a moderate-sized hospital might expect to generate a half-million-dollar surplus per year (Dorazio 1984; paraphrased).

Developing a strategy for controlling the health care system, with its web of contracts and regulatory and reimbursement mechanisms, has been a major goal of public policy ever since the passage of Medicare and Medicaid legislation. How can policy makers control cost increases, eliminate substandard care, and assure reasonable access? System controls rely on the same power strategies used by provider organizations to control their members. Such power may be coercive, such as naming a special prosecutor to investigate fraud and abuse; remunerative, such as negotiating contracts with third-party financing organizations; or normative, such as meeting standards of professional accrediting bodies. While in principle a variety of control strategies is possible, many policy makers believe that they promise more than they can deliver. Efforts to redress the inadequacies of system controls fall into two general categories: regulatory and market.

The rationale of the regulatory approach is simple: control the number of providers, what you pay them, and the nature of the product they deliver, and you control the system. The power to exert such control depends on the ability to curtail public funding, revoke licensure to operate, or impose legal sanctions for noncompliance. While authority is not open-ended and is certainly subject to judicial review, the legislative and executive branches of both state and federal governments have the power to impose and enforce such controls (American Hospital Association 1985).

Upon close examination, however, it is often unclear who is controlling whom. First, restricting the number of providers of services increases society's dependency on them and, consequently, increases their power. If health facilities have only enough beds and services to provide for immediate needs, no facility can be allowed to go bankrupt or can even be shut down for providing substandard care without threatening the health of the very population that the regulatory bodies are supposed to be protecting. In essence, the providers hold the population hostage. Second, controlling prices does not necessarily control providers. Providers can choose not to participate. Indeed, this has been a perennial problem with physician participation in the Medicaid program and with access to nursing homes for Medicaid patients. The Medicaid program pays higher costs for the hospitalization of patients denied admission to nursing homes. Participating outpatient providers can also "game" the pricing system by "pingponging" patients; that is, a routine office visit is transformed into a variety of additional procedures and services, which may include supplying eyeglasses and orthopedic shoes for every family member that accompanies the patient.

Clearly, power in this situation is not unilateral. The political repercussions are felt by any regulatory body that forces an institution into bankruptcy; thus a fine line must be walked to avoid an appeal process or prolonged negotiations or both. On this front, providers have a clear advantage. Just as the Internal Revenue Service serves as the training ground for corporate tax lawyers, so state rate-setting groups serve as educational institutions for providers and provider associations. As a result, rate-setting groups have high turnover and relatively young, inexperienced staff members facing experienced negotiating teams that have far more resources. In one case involving a new nursing home chain, state regulatory bodies found themselves up against the former director of the agency that licensed nursing homes in the state, the former state director of health planning, the individual responsible for developing the Medicaid reimbursement system in the state, a former nursing home auditor, and a former nursing home inspector (Ganey 1978, 1).

The regulatory body must oversee many providers, and it generally has inadequate staff and limited resources to allocate to any particular case. It prefers not to be driven into a protracted appeal process in the courts. The provider has a clear, immediate financial stake in the outcome and controls access to the information upon which the merits of the case are judged. Accommodation, if not outright co-optation, becomes the norm (McClure 1981). In New York State, for example, the rate of increase in Medicaid payments to nursing homes has followed a four-year cycle. The peak is reached in the gubernatorial election year, which usually corresponds to the contract negotiating period between nursing homes and the union representing their employees (Smith 1981, 89). New wage concessions are passed through the Medicaid reimbursement formulas for nursing homes. The workers get their wage increase, the governor gets some votes for his reelection bid (since the wage hike impact on taxes will not show up until after the election), and the nursing home operators are left unaffected. Thus, one set of social-legal contracts dovetails with another.

The alternative is to allow the "invisible hand"—the law of supply and demand—to control providers. The free market, many persons argue, as a regulator is more efficient and more responsive to consumers than the government is (McClure 1981, Havighurst 1976, Ellwood 1974). There is, indeed, much magic that can be worked by the invisible hand. Fifteen years ago, for example, it was virtually impossible within licensed settings for a father to attend the birth of his children. Today, hospitals in most major metropolitan areas take out full-page newspaper ads extolling their family-centered services, including full participation by the husband in the delivery, rooming in, flexible visiting hours, homelike birthing rooms, and even free candelight surf and turf, champagne dinners for the parents (McNaughton 1981). It is no accident that these changes took place in a period of declining birth rates (and, consequently, declining occupancy rates in hospital maternity units), which forced greater competition among hospitals. Ten years ago, the kind of contracts that radiologists negotiated with hospitals provoked public outrage. Today those contracts are far tighter and less lucrative in many areas. The change came about more because of the increase in the number of radiologists in relation to the number of available hospital positions than because of public outrage.

Do such market-produced changes really address the control problems of cost, quality, access, and equity? The hospitals, in head-to-head competition with each other for maternity admissions, still have to deal with costs of excess capacity as well as costs associated with aggressive marketing of these services. One way or another, at least in the short run, while there is still competition, these costs will be passed on. When competition dwindles, what will happen to the advantages that accrue from it? Radiologists, unhappy with or unable to obtain hospital contracts, have gone into business for themselves in some areas of the country. While prices per unit of service will no doubt drop as a result, the overall number of units of service will jump dramatically, as will, probably, overall costs.

Will the invisible hand improve the quality of services? One condition necessary for the competitive model to work—adequate information—is lacking in most patients' decisions about health services. The social contract between provider and patient gives the provider the power to make decisions in the patient's best interest. Many persons are loath to undermine the social contract, even though the competitive model fails to take into account the externalities, or benefits, that accrue to the larger community from the services received by an individual (that is, reduction of the costs of communicable diseases, costs to the community resulting from premature death or disability of an individual, and so on). What is appropriate at the individual provider-patient level is at least as appropriate at the system level. Should the health care system, like the individual provider, provide only those services that are profitable, ignoring what can improve the health of the population? Who should provide services for the poorest and sickest segments of the population (which are now the least profitable)? If competition will not serve the overall health needs of a population, how will society fill the gap? Should the health care system provide surf and turf dinners to new parents and eliminate prenatal care for the urban poor? Should the health care system provide three-dimensional color pictures of sinus headaches at convenient locations in shopping malls instead of adequate emergency services? The more health care is viewed as an economic good and the less it is viewed as a social relationship or professional service, the more likely it is that the answers to such questions will be yes.

As definitions of health care change, so do distribution of power, sources of power, and structure of the system itself. These changes, in turn, have shifted the way individuals and organizations are controlled and influenced. The sense of shared mission is evaporating, and with it the atmosphere of trust that enables individuals to work toward common goals. The sense of mission is being replaced with tighter external controls and a far more adversarial relationship between parties. Figure 6.3 summarizes what this change has meant in terms of organizational relationships within the system and the patterns of control imposed upon providers. Changes have transformed the environmental control mechanism from what was essentially a normative structure to one that is increasingly adversarial and coercive.

CONCLUSIONS

These adversarial struggles have changed the structure of the system and, consequently, the relative power of various participants. The changes, which have been particularly dramatic in the last 25 years, were described in some detail in chapter 1. Briefly summarized, they are as follows:

1. Size: a dramatic increase in the average size of facilities providing services, including hospitals, nursing homes, and office practices
2. Specialization: increased specialization in the provision of services by individual providers, departments within organizations, and facilities
3. Centralization: increased centralization of control, reflected in the development of multi-institutional systems through mergers, acquisitions, or expansion of satellite services by hospitals, nursing homes, even medical practices

Figure 6.3   Qualitative Shifts in Patterns of Control of Health Care Providers

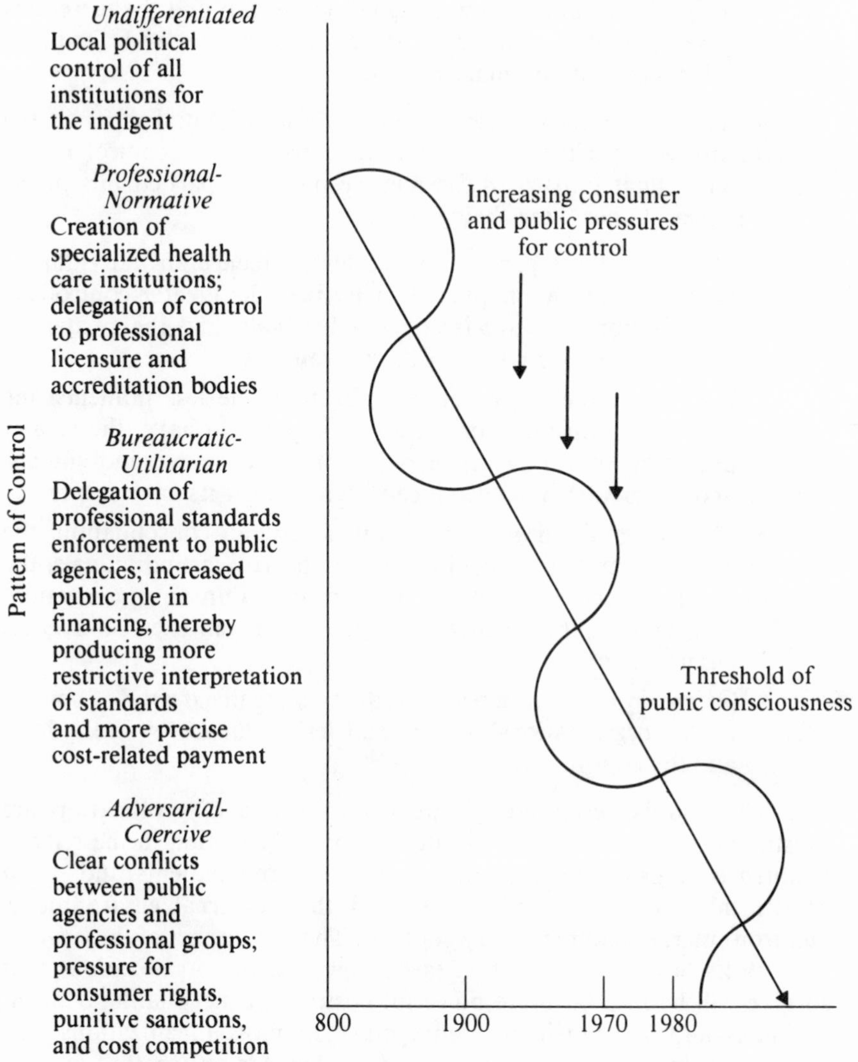

Undifferentiated
Local political control of all institutions for the indigent

*Professional-
Normative*
Creation of specialized health care institutions; delegation of control to professional licensure and accreditation bodies

*Bureaucratic-
Utilitarian*
Delegation of professional standards enforcement to public agencies; increased public role in financing, thereby producing more restrictive interpretation of standards and more precise cost-related payment

*Adversarial-
Coercive*
Clear conflicts between public agencies and professional groups; pressure for consumer rights, punitive sanctions, and cost competition

Pattern of Control

Increasing consumer and public pressures for control

Threshold of public consciousness

800   1900   1970 1980

Source: Smith 1982, 124.

4. Privatization: more frequent governance of health facilities by private for-profit structures, reflected in the development of for-profit hospital and nursing home systems and the increasing development of similarly structured private and for-profit subsidiaries of voluntary facilities

While it is not entirely clear whether these structural shifts caused or were caused by changes in the general patterns of control in the health sector, their impact on the relative power of participants in the system is clear. Other things being equal:

1. The larger the organization, the less influence an individual is likely to have in shaping its activities, the greater control the organization can exercise over individuals, and the greater influence it can exercise over its environment.

2. The higher the degree of specialization, the less influence the individual consumer or employee is likely to have, the greater degree of control the organization can exercise over individuals, and the greater influence it can exercise over its environment.

3. The higher the degree of centralization and consolidation, the greater control the organization can exert over individuals, the less influence individuals can exercise within an organization, and the greater influence the organization can exercise over its environment.

4. Greater private ownership produces a greater degree of control by the organizations' leaders and less influence by individuals and the community.

These shifts, produced by bureaucratization and privatization, are illustrated in figure 6.4. They result in a major reduction in the relativeinfluence of professionals, other employees, and patients and much greater insulation of organizations from their external environments and from market and regulatory controls. The full impact of these structural shifts has yet to be felt. Clearly, however, the organizations that survive will be in a far more powerful position for negotiating with individuals and with their environments than most organizations currently in existence. Is this good or bad? It depends on whether one defines medical care as an economic good, a professional service, or a social relationship. It also depends on whether one (and the organizations) perceives power in this context as a fixed or an expandable resource.

Figure 6.4   Trends That Enhance the Power of Health Services Organizations

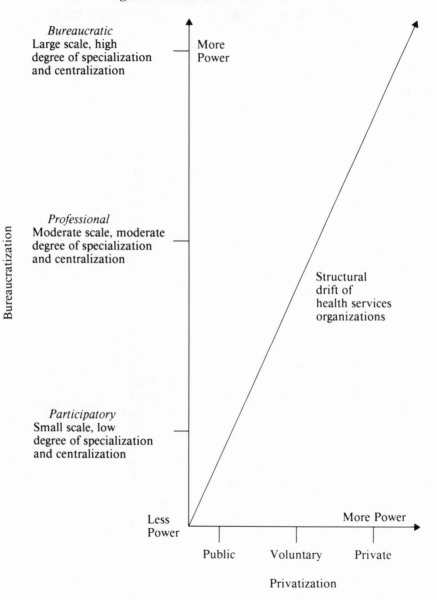

In the final section of this book, we will look at: the process by which these and related changes have taken and will take place; the strategies that will be used by various actors; and the relative merits for the health care system of alternative structures.

Part

III

Escaping the Labyrinth

7

Paths

It would be an unsound fancy and
self-contradictory to expect that things
which have never yet been done can be done except
by means which have never been tried.

Francis Bacon
The New Organon

In the first section of this book we described the various parts of the labyrinth and how they were assembled; in the second, the underlying physical and behavioral mechanisms that govern its operation. In this final section we describe how to escape the constraints of the labyrinth to do things that have never been done by means that have never been tried.

One can choose how to operate the health care system and what to attempt to accomplish with it. In this chapter we describe alternative ways in which to accomplish things that have never been done. In chapter 8 we describe what tactics an individual can use to influence outcomes, and in the final chapter we describe what outcomes can be achieved.

As we suggested in chapter 4, organizations respond to pressure to change by searching for solutions that require limited effort to find and minimal disruption of the status quo. Figure 7.1 summarizes this process. Changes produced by a search I require only minor repackaging and innovations in the public relations efforts of the organization, but nothing else. Search II changes require improvements in existing operations and practices. Most articles in the trade magazines for health providers bring such innovations to their attention. Search III changes re-

Figure 7.1 Organizational Response to Pressure to Change

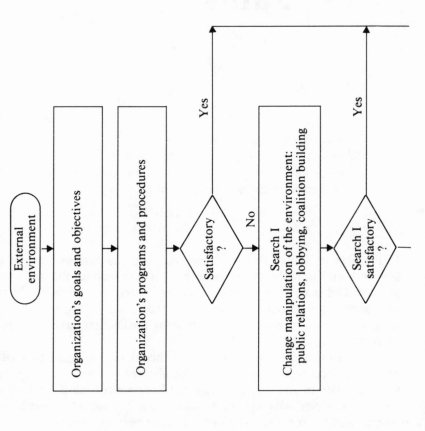

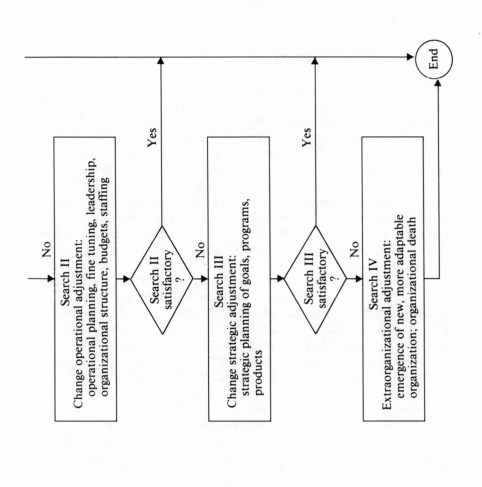

quire a far more involved and disruptive response; an organization must alter its goals and its services. Search IV changes involve the actual disappearance of the existing organizational structure and the creation of new forms. It is in the search IV direction, the doing of things that have never been done by means that have never been tried, that we are headed.

SOURCES OF CHANGE

Organizations and systems change in response to different kinds of pressure. Change may be the result of internal pressures generated by members who are dissatisfied with performance, or it may be the result of external pressure generated by elements in the environment that influence performance. Like individuals, organizations or systems can be described as inner-directed or other-directed. Hospitals connected with medical schools tend to respond to the demands of their faculty, often at the expense of patients and of the hospital's ability to generate income from third-party payers. Many of the more successful for-profit firms, on the other hand, are other-directed, or market-driven, making very self-conscious, carefully thought-out decisions about where to locate, what services to provide, and when to buy, sell, or close facilities.

There is a fine line between an open organization (or an open-minded individual) and an empty organization (or empty-minded individual). An organization that becomes too inner-directed suffers the organizational equivalent of autism, and its ability to survive is put at risk. On the other hand, an organization that becomes too other- or market-directed loses its ability to structure and control events and is forced into an entirely reactive position. Most organizations try to balance the two. For example, six out of the eight "patrician elite" medical school hospitals in the East had become involved in the establishment of for-profit subsidiaries, preferred provider organizations (PPOs), HMOs, or other such market-oriented activities by the end of 1983, in spite of their long tradition of aloofness to such endeavors. At a meeting of medical school deans, an informal poll indicated that the majority of them had been discussing possible business ventures with for-profit corporations (Relman 1984, 22). Similarly, some of the larger for-profit hospital corporations have been involved in efforts to acquire or become affiliated with research and teaching facilities—and to develop experimental artificial heart programs—in an effort to move away from a completely reactive, other-directed position.

Change may result from planned or unplanned efforts. The advantage of planned change is that it tries to balance these two orientations.

However, like the champion downhill skier, successful organizations and those who manage them can never be fully in control.

Anyone who follows the sport will remember the fantastic run of Franz Klammer in the Men's Downhill in the 1976 Winter Olympics. He seemed "out of control" for the entire run, which in skiing language means he was on the verge of falling and in fact looked as though he surely would fall throughout the entire run. He did not fall and won the Olympic Gold Medal. Up until Klammer's run the prevailing thinking among downhill racers was that the winner of a race would be the one who was in the best condition, had the best technique, and skied just this side of the edge of losing control. By the time the 1980 Winter Olympics came the thinking had changed. Now, the thinking is that to win a race one has to ski on the other side of the edge of losing control— that is, one must ski out of control and hope to avoid a fall by recovering from being too much out of control. In 1976 Klammer was the only one (of the truly world-class skiers) who skied out of control, and since every other top skier was trying to ski just short of losing control, Klammer won easily. Now all top skiers, perhaps fifteen or twenty, are skiing out of control and on any given day it is largely natural selection stemming from factors beyond the skier's control which determines who wins. During any run there are many blind variations in the form of ruts, bumps, mistakes, and so forth, which are all beyond the control of the skiers at the speed they are now going. The skier who skis most out of control and is luckiest in avoiding falling will win. Each skier knows that he cannot determine his winning just by training, good technique, and skiing at the edge of control. But skiing out of control only guarantees he will have to make numerous miraculous recoveries from near falls. The skier who takes the most risks and makes the most miraculous recoveries wins. The skier who skis in control does have control over his destiny and guarantees only one thing—losing. Since there are so many good skiers skiing out of control the odds are excellent that one of them will always take enough risks and manage enough miraculous recoveries to beat the under-control skier (McKelvey 1982, 447–48).

Table 7.1 summarizes the planned and unplanned, internal and external sources of pressure to change. These four sources have shaped the changes in health services organization that we described in detail in the first two sections of this book. For illustrative purposes, we have

Table 7.1 Sources of Pressure to Change

Search	Internal Pressure		External Pressure	
	Planned	Unplanned	Planned	Unplanned
Search I: environmental manipulation (example: family-centered maternity care)	Public relations (Promotion of obstetric services)	Informal networks (Obstetric and nursing staff advocacy)	Pro forma regulation (Health planning agency's imposition of volume and occupancy requirements)	Shifting consumer preferences (Childbirth education movement)
Search II: operational adjustment (example: acquisition of nuclear magnetic resonance, NMR)	Operational, tactical planning (Planned expansion of existing services)	Staff coalitions (Medical staff pressure for state-of-the-art equipment)	Altered third-party or government regulations (Third-party decisions concerning reimbursement of service for particular diagnoses)	Market shifts and technical breakthroughs (Refinement of NMR technology; evaluation of diagnostic efficacy)

Search III: strategic planning (example: satellite ambulatory surgery)	Strategic planning (Strategic diversification)	Altered ruling coalition (Pressure from staff to increase surgical capacity)	Major legislative initiatives (DRG reimbursement increases profitability of ambulatory surgery)	Major political and economic shifts (Creation of preferred provider organizations by business groups; increased HMO market share)
Search IV: extra-organizational adjustment (example: consolidation of facility into multi-institutional system)	Corporate restructuring (Planned strategic response to financial exigencies)	Unanticipated financial exigencies (Threatened bankruptcy or inability to raise capital for facility replacement)	Cataclysmic shifts in public policy (Payment freeze and retroactive denial of payments)	Major social and economic upheaval (Serious recession)

included an example of a change that was influenced by pressures from each of these sources at each of the four search levels described in figure 7.1. For example, search I efforts to change the packaging of maternity services have been subjected to pressures produced by (1) changes in public expectations brought about by the childbirth education movement, (2) health services planning agency requirements for certain occupancy rates for hospital maternity services, (3) changes in the attitudes of the hospital's nurses and obstetricians, and (4) conscious efforts on the part of hospital management to improve obstetric occupancy rates by promoting family-centered maternity services. Search II efforts to acquire a nuclear magnetic resonance scanner have often been the result of (1) the rapid refinement of this technology, (2) the decision of third parties to reimburse such services, (3) support for the acquisition from staff physicians, and (4) the planned expansion of radiological services. Search III efforts to establish a satellite ambulatory surgery center have often been stimulated by (1) the threat of competitive, independently owned PPOs or HMOs, (2) disincentives to treat certain surgical cases on an inpatient basis (produced by the shift to a DRG payment system), (3) demands from the surgical staff for expanded capacity, and (4) strategic planning efforts on the part of board and management to assure the institution's survival through diversification. Search IV changes that result in the facility's absorption into a larger, multi-institutional system might be triggered by (1) financial pressures on providers and third parties produced by a serious recession, (2) excessively restrictive changes in third-party payment, (3) staff dissatisfaction with the facility's resources, or (4) the planning efforts of the facility's management.

Much emphasis has been placed recently on strategic, market-oriented, tactical planning. The buzz words used to describe these activites change every six months, but the emphasis is on reducing the uncertainty an organization faces by actively seeking solutions. Some of these planned activities have resulted in radical restructuring. Sometimes, like the downhill skiers, such efforts go out of control and still fail to win the race. According to some consultants, the bulk of their more recent business has involved the undoing of these ill-fated voyages into new corporate and organizational forms (Steinberg 1984). Unplanned pressure for change, such as shifts in the ruling coalition within an organization or in the regulatory environment, can have a far greater impact on how organizations change than all the most carefully structured plans.

PATHWAY OF CHANGE

No matter how planned or unplanned, extensive or limited, change follows a predictable pathway, summarized in figure 7.2. The first stage is the *recognition of a problem* by organizational participants who perceive a gap between what the organization is currently doing and what it should, could, or must do (Downs 1967). This recognition may be sparked internally, by the expectations of participants, or externally, by community or regulatory pressures to expand or restrict existing programs and activities. The second stage, *identification of an innovation*, signals agreement by decision makers as to the appropriate way to narrow the gap between actual and desired performance. The third stage, *implementation of the innovation*, involves putting in place the changes agreed upon by the decision makers. Implementation, however, provides no guarantee that the change will survive: it must stand the test of time and be adopted and accepted by those responsible for using it. This final stage, *institutionalization of the innovation*, is often the major stumbling block for change. The road to successful institutionalization is rarely short or smooth.

Organizational characteristics can facilitate or impede the passage of an innovation through the four stages. We will look at the evidence and then try to reach some conclusions about the impact that bureaucratic, professional, and participatory structures have on this process.

Stage 1: Recognition of a Problem

As suggested by figure 7.2, recognition of a problem can be generated externally or internally. In either case, it depends on pressure for change generated by a discrepancy between organizational performance and expectations of what the organization should or could do.

While it is generally accepted that the external environment has a significant impact on stage 1, it may affect the organization in different ways. One view is that health care organizations add service and technology in response to local needs or professional logic (Kaluzny et al. 1971, Warner 1975, Russell 1979). Another view is that organizations add technology in order to protect themselves against liability. For example, as hospitals are being held to an increasingly rigorous standard of performance by external accreditation agencies and legal requirements, technologies of questionable quality and reliability are being added, not to enhance performance, but to demonstrate the hospitals' good intentions should they be sued (McNeil and Miniham 1977).

Figure 7.2   The Process of Innovation

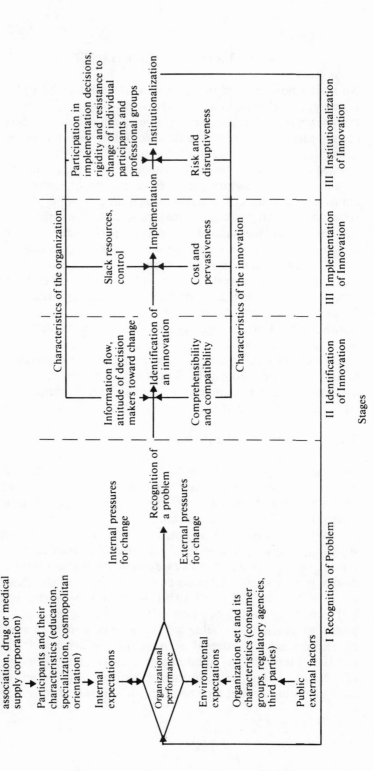

The greater the specialization of participants in an organization, the more likely they are to recognize a potential problem. While the diversity resulting from specialization and the conflicting aspirations of specialists are difficult to accommodate, the number of specialties and the relation of those specialties to administrators and trustees are positively correlated with the number of new programs and costly technologies adopted. For example, coalitions of hospital-based specialists, business-oriented administrators, and trustees supporting technological expansion as a competitive strategy exert considerable pressure for hospitals to acquire new, expensive technology (Greer 1984).

The characteristics of individuals are also likely to be important during stage 1. The more cosmopolitan their orientation—that is, the greater their awareness of and interest in what is going on in similar institutions—the more likely participants are to perceive a gap between what their own institution is doing and what it could or should be doing. Innovations that are more politically controversial and less professionally respectable are likely to be implemented in departments staffed by less professional, less cosmopolitan health officers, and vice versa (Becker 1970). Less cosmopolitan individuals tend to be more responsive to local needs and less concerned with what their professional peers are doing. In general, the more cosmopolitan and well trained the staff within the organization, the more likely they are to recognize performance gaps. (Kaluzny, Veney, and Gentry 1974, Mohr 1969, Mytinger 1968, Kaplan 1967).

Of course, only staff members who are aware of what is happening within their institutions can get upset about performance. Hospitals' implementation of new medical technology for the treatment of respiratory diseases, for example, has been found to be positively related to the existence of tissue committees, medical record committees, internal medical audits, and involvement in clinical research (Morse, Gordon, and Moch 1974).

Stage 2: Identification of an Innovation

Once key decision makers have recognized a problem, they search for a solution. In general, they prefer to import a prepackaged solution rather than engage in costly internal research and development (Pelz and Munson 1982). The search proceeds through the levels described in figure 7.1 until a satisfactory solution is found. The better equipped (in terms of staff resources and general orientation) an organization is to search for solutions, the more thorough those searches are likely to be (Kimberly 1978). Participants need to gather and evaluate information and make inquiries of other institutions likely to have similar problems. More effective communication within an organization is also likely to enhance the search process and lead to the identification of an appropriate innovation. For example, the frequency of informal communication among personnel of a social service agency appears to be positively related to innovation (Hage 1974). Such cross-fertilization seems to facilitate identification of innovations by organizational decision makers. Similarly, greater mutual understanding of the problems faced by administrators, medical staff, and trustees helps facilitate the process of change.

If a change can be easily described, if its consequences are easily understood, and if it is compatible with the existing orientation of the institution, organizational decision makers are likely to implement it. Thus technological changes, or hardware, tend to fare better than more abstract programs and ideas, or software (Pelz and Munson 1980). It is possible to touch technological changes and to see what they do. Such innovations are also compatible with the professional orientation of physicians, which dominates most hospitals and other health care organizations.

Depending on their attitudes, decision makers may either embrace an innovative alternative or cling to the status quo. Predictably, more positive administrative attitudes toward change have been found to be related to higher rates of innovation (Mohr 1971). Similarly, more positive attitudes toward change among board members of social service agencies have been found to be related to higher rates of innovation (Hooyman and Kaplan 1976). A particularly potent indicator of high rates of innovation appears to be the combination of positive attitudes toward change among administrators and among other elite participants in organizational decisions (Hage and Dewar 1973). This appears to be particularly important with more social, less technological innovations, such as childbirth education classes as opposed to fetal monitors (Nathanson and Morlock 1980).

Stage 3: Implementation of the Innovation

Implementation of an innovation depends on the nature of the innovation, the resources available to implement it, and the control the decision makers can exercise over its implementation. Less costly innovations, in terms of manpower and financial resources, and those that affect only part of an organization can be implemented more easily. New drugs and relatively inexpensive medical equipment can be adopted rapidly, whereas more costly and pervasive changes, such as the reorganization of the medical staff, may take years in the recognition and identification stages alone (Kaluzny and Veney 1977).

Ease of implementation depends on the characteristics of the innovation and the type of organization (Downs and Mohr 1979). Hospitals will implement health service programs relatively easily if the programs can be shown to enhance revenues and expand the comprehensiveness of their services. Public health departments, on the other hand, seem more likely to implement programs that are consistent with their preventive orientation and that can be implemented on a small-scale trial basis. Evidently public health departments are less concerned about the overall comprehensiveness of the services they provide and are rarely concerned about generating revenue (Kaluzny, Veney, and Gentry 1974).

Certain innovations may be linked in such a way that implementation of one tends to facilitate implementation of the others. For example, the implementation of insurance coverage of treatment programs for alcoholism facilitates the implementation of the treatment program itself (Fennell 1984). Similarly, implementation of a computerized medical records system is a prerequisite to the successful implementation of a quality assurance program (Kaluzny 1982).

Uncommitted manpower and resources help facilitate the implementation of more costly innovations. If a financial surplus exists and if staff members do not have enough to do in terms of day-to-day operations, then a way will be found to spend the money and occupy staff time by implementing a new program. Much of the recent explosion in organizational and program innovation in hospitals is related to the overall increase in the size of administrative staff and the creation of planning and marketing positions.

Prospective reimbursement systems tend to limit slack time and money and, therefore, the implementation of innovations (Cromwell and Kanak 1982). Recent analysis suggests, however, that the implementation of cost-saving innovations may be enhanced by prospective reimbursement systems. In a study of six states, three with prospective reimbursement and three without, researchers found a decrease in the implementation of cost-increasing technology (such as electronic fetal monitoring and volumetric infusion pumps) and an increase in the implementation of cost-saving innovations (such as automated bacterial susceptibility testing and centralized energy management systems) (Romeo, Wagner, and Lee 1984).

The type of control within the organization may either facilitate or impede implementation, depending on the characteristics of the innovation. For example, rules and regulations compatible with the attributes of the innovation tend to facilitate its implementation (Scheirer 1981). Similarly, narrowly defined job descriptions and licensure laws that prescribe what various occupational groups can and cannot do hamper all but the least imaginative innovations. The director of an outpatient clinic set up by a local health department expresses the frustration that imaginative and concerned participants feel in such situations:

> The trouble with this organization is that there is just too much red tape—*of course* we need new programs that help the department to relate better to the community. But we do things by the book here—and before I can get a Spanish-speaking nurse and indigenous workers, we need to develop and change job descriptions as well as increase the number of positions allocated to this particular unit—and you know how long that takes! The problem is not here, but with those idiots in the state capital who sit around adding pages to the rule manuals.

Very formal organizational structure is an obstacle to rapid implementation. The implementation of new drugs (Rosner 1968), pulmonary technology (Morse, Gordon, and Moch 1974), and health care programs (Kaluzny, Veney, and Gentry 1974, Palumbo 1969, Hage and Aiken 1967) has been shown to be adversely affected by formality. Implementation is also likely to be slowed if members of an organization lack clear guidelines for dealing with new programs or technologies. In other words, given a recognized problem and an identified solution, persons within an organization that lets them know what they are supposed to do will generally do it.

In highly differentiated organizations, decentralized decision making facilitates the implementation of innovations that are compatible with the functional units of the organization (Moch and Morse 1977). Innovations that affect several different units, however, are more easily implemented when there is greater central control to prevent departments or individuals from splintering off and rejecting them. This control may take many forms, such as permanent interdepartmental coordinating committees and temporary interdepartmental teams to resolve specific problems.

Stage 4: Institutionalization of the Innovation

Acceptance of the implemented innovation is the final hurdle. Most organizations have implemented innovations that died from disuse or as a result of the hostility or indifference of those responsible for their day-to-day care. A service unit management program is abandoned after six months. A home care program is established by a hospital but is eventually terminated because physicians fail to refer patients to it. A medical information system is implemented, yet the procedures in the previous manual continue to be used. Such innovations fail to become institutionalized because of the way decisions were made to implement them, because of the attitudes and behavior of the individuals entrusted with their care, and because of the characteristics of the innovations themselves. Participation in decision making results in greater commitment to an innovation. Individuals are less likely to ignore or abuse one that they helped implement in the first place.

Personal characteristics may predispose individuals to accept implemented innovations. For example, in a study of medical information systems (Kjerulff 1982, Kjerulff et al. 1983), researchers found that hospital personnel with more positive attitudes toward change had less difficulty using a new system. Role ambiguity, job mobility, and work shift were associated with difficulty in using a new system. Work shift was particularly critical. The day shift reported more difficulty than other shifts, partly because of numerous breakdowns and partly because of less opportunity to experiment with the system and learn to incorporate it into work roles.

The individual's position in the larger communication network of the organization is also a significant factor. Analysis of physician use of hospital information systems shows that physicians who are more socially integrated into the network tend to be early adopters and that cohesive groups of physicians were likely to have similar attitudes toward the innovation and to adopt it at about the same time (Anderson and Jay 1985).

Failure to attract or allocate sufficient resources and failure to resolve conflict among personnel are frequently cited reasons for terminating implemented innovations. A study of implemented unit management systems found a failure rate of approximately 20 percent. Insufficient financial resources, inability to attract qualified managerial personnel, and sustained conflict between unit managers and clinical personnel were factors leading to termination of the systems (Burns 1982).

THE PROCESS OF CHANGE
IN THREE KINDS OF ORGANIZATIONS

Different kinds of organizations recognize different problems and identify, implement, and institutionalize quite different kinds of change. We can demonstrate this fact by describing how the process works in three different kinds of organizations, each with a different definition of health care.

Health Care As an Economic Good:
The For-Profit Hospital Chain

For-profit hospital chains are concerned with growth and returns to their stockholders. They tend to be centrally controlled and subject to industrial rationality. Indexes of organizational efficiency, such as staffing ratios, occupancy rates, and bad debts, are carefully monitored. When performance on such indices is compared among various hospitals in the system, the consequences of any "inefficiencies" are immediately visible and lead to investigation. The search for solutions is facilitated by a skilled, well-trained, central research and development staff. Since the same standardized "solutions" can be applied to all hospitals, individual hospitals, with limited staff, do not have to reinvent the wheel. If a change can enhance revenues, awareness of that change is rapidly translated into implementation.

Because strong central control enables rapid implementation, control is maintained by essentially buying physicians out from any substantial involvement in the structuring of the system and by militantly opposing employee unions. Both actions assure that the managerial prerogatives of executives are not infringed. Whatever self-selection or organizational selection in staffing may occur helps in the institutionalization of such changes. As a result, for-profit hospital chains have apparently been substantially more profitable than their nonprofit counterparts. Because they exploit the third-party payment system more effectively than many nonprofit community hospitals, for-profit chains have been able to provide a healthy return on investments and plow a good deal of money back into their systems. They have led the way in modular construction of facilities and in efforts to automate various operations. In terms of efficiency, for-profit hospital chains have been by far the most innovative organizations in the field of health care.

Health Care As a Professional Relationship:
The University Hospital

The university teaching hospital attempts to be the model for technical excellence. It is the professional training ground for those who will eventually staff other institutions. Activities of all practitioners are carefully monitored, and medical records and tissue review committees, as well as other technical quality review mechanisms, provide systematic surveillance and ensure visibility of the quality of care provided. A university hospital is a highly complex operation built around a bewildering variety of practitioners and staff specialists, each with a highly developed area of expertise and a strong desire to see that expertise used by the institution. Ongoing research efforts within the institution continually ask basic questions about treatment procedures. As a result of these concerns, and the visibility surrounding them, such an institution is unlikely to be satisfied with its technical performance in any area. The search for alternative solutions in terms of medical research is a part of routine operation. Desirable technical innovations can be identified rapidly, because this research is carried out close to the day-to-day operations of the institution.

The highly decentralized departmental structure of university hospitals aids in the implementation of technological change, within boundaries. While a more centralized control structure would prevent rapid adoption of new techniques or procedures, the autonomy given professional departments facilitates rapid adoption.

Because decision making at the departmental level is generally collegial in nature, most of the individuals who will use a technological change are directly involved in the decision to implement it. Hence, the innovation is easily institutionalized. Professional commitment to the advancement of medical treatment also fosters acceptance of innovations. Almost by definition, university hospitals are innovative in improving the technical quality of care.

**Health Care As a Social Relationship:
The Innovative, Small-Town Community Hospital**

Ten years ago, the hospital faced a crisis. Declining occupancy, an aging medical staff, and a deteriorating physical plant threatened its survival. The new highway put institutions in the adjacent urban center only 30 minutes away. The hospital's financial condition was aggravated by its obligation to provide a large percentage of free care, since many persons in the community lacked health insurance. It could not compete by providing health care as an economic (profitable) good or as a professional (technically most advanced) service. Its immediate options were either to close or to become a satellite of one of the hospitals in the urban center.

The community's opposition to these options sparked a resurgence of interest in the hospital. A series of community meetings began a profound process of organizational renewal. New members were added to the board to assure a greater sense of community ownership. A shared vision of the hospital as a community resource, one that provided a broad range of services, emerged. The fate of the community and the hospital became linked. The hospital became an important part of the community development strategy, adding to the attractiveness of the community as a residential area for those working in the urban center and as a site for relocation of service industries and small manufacturing plants. It was also recognized that, in order to compete with the hospitals in the urban center, the hospital had to do a better job not only of assuring high-quality care but also of ensuring that care was provided in a far more pleasant way to patients.

A new administrator assisted in the renewal of the hospital. He successfully recruited physicians, most of whom had just completed their family practice residency, and assisted in the establishment of their practices. These new physicians became actively involved in developing preventive education programs, home care, an outpatient alcohol program, and rehabilitation services that fit in with the new vision of the hospital and the imperatives for its survival. At least as important in the revitalization of the hospital was the involvement of the nursing and other staff. Their livelihoods were also dependent on the hospital's survival, and they were willing and active participants in hospital team meetings. They were quick to identify both problems and innovations that would improve the hospital's ability to respond to the needs of its patients.

The new facility, which housed the new programs as well as the traditional hospital services, embodied the revitalized vision of the hospital and the participation of community members and staff. It was built on a beautifully landscaped campus with a view of the lake and stood in stark contrast to the old building. It boasted gourmet cuisine, candlelight dinners, and wine. Family members were encouraged to be actively involved in the treatment of patients, and rooming-in arrangements were available in most patient rooms.

Hospital volunteers provided stereo cassettes and videotapes in their new patient library in addition to books. Like the staff, the volunteers were quick to point out problems related to the amenities of patient care. Since many of them were related to board members, these problems usually received prompt attention.

Somewhere in this process, in part because of the organizational renewal efforts and in part because of the growth of the population and the increasingly wealthy, suburban flavor of the town, the tables turned. The community hospital ceased to be a supplicant and was actively wooed by the urban specialists and tertiary-care hospitals. In exchange for backup specialty services, the hospital was able to impose the same standards of consumer responsiveness on these providers that it imposed on itself. Failure to consistently live up to these standards would jeopardize the continuation of referral arrangements. This, too, was an innovative organization.

CONCLUSIONS

Various factors affect an innovation's chances of success or failure. The more visible an organization's problems are, the more likely it is that something will be done about them. A newspaper story about the inadequacy of the emergency room may spark action. A health systems agency report documenting the need for support services for the elderly poor may generate action within a public health department. An analysis by the tissue committee showing that a high percentage of normal appendixes had been removed may cause anger and corrective action within a hospital's medical staff. The truth is always friendly, but it takes strong and committed administrators and professional staff members to see it that way.

The kinds of individuals hired by an organization will affect its ability to recognize problems. The hiring of new individuals with more specialized skills or different perspectives will uncover problems that were overlooked previously.

Once a problem is recognized, the ability to identify a solution will be affected by how easy it is to get information and how people responsible for making decisions feel about changes. The more information and concrete facts that can be supplied about an innovation (that is, the less uncertainty about how to implement it and what its impact will be), the more likely it is to be selected. The more willing decision makers are to innovate and experiment with new procedures and programs, the less evidence and information will be required and the more quickly an innovation will be identified.

How the innovation is presented will also influence its identification and adoption. It needs to be easy to understand and to appear compatible with the values and orientation of the persons adopting it. Prepaid group practices languished as somewhat questionable, even socialistic schemes in the 1930s, but when they were repackaged as health maintenance organizations, designed to encourage competition and, consequently, cost containment in the health care sector, they took off. Diagnosis-related groups were an obscure research tool for classifying the use patterns of hospitals until a similar simplification and repackaging took place.

Implementing change requires some slack in resources and the ability to alter the structure of an organization. Changes that can first be implemented on a small scale, with little initial impact on an organization, have a better chance of survival. Medicare reimbursement on the basis of DRGs, for example, was first implemented on an experimental basis.

Institutionalizing an innovation often requires further persuasion and change in attitudes. If the innovation can be packaged to require few adjustments and changes in work patterns and no risk to the individuals concerned (that they might be laid off or lose income), it will be more easily accepted. The development of independent practice associations in the last 20 years, for example, has dramatically altered local medical society and physician resistance to HMOs.

More specific tactics for facilitating movement along the path to institutionalization are described in the next chapter.

8

Tactics

The least satisfying thing about my job is that the changes that are needed just don't happen. Getting anything accomplished in this place is like moving a graveyard. Even the most obvious, simplest things take forever. You have to keep pushing and persuading, even when it seems like everybody would gain from it. Then when you do get something changed, there's no guarantee it won't be sabotaged and die from disuse and neglect. You have to have the tenacity of a bulldog and the time perspective of a turtle to cope with it.

Hospital administrator

The process of moving the system can be slow and exhausting, and it is easy to become disheartened. Our discussions of institutional inertia, however, were designed to provide a realistic appraisal of the task rather than to cast a shadow of gloom over the possibilities. Change does take place, and graveyards do get moved. Sometimes it is useful to remember how things were in the past.

Change in the Treatment
of Children in Hospitals

In the early 1950's Children's Medical Center in Boston was involved in a ground breaking experiment. An attempt was made to measure the effect of traditional hospital procedures, as opposed to more consciously designed, emotionally supportive ones, on their patients. The "experimental" group was allowed daily visiting by parents during several hours each day, early ambulation where possible, a special play program employing a nursery school teacher, and other forms of psychological preparation and support by the professional staff. Parents of these patients were also allowed to accompany their children to the ward to meet the staff and to assist in their initial adjustment. The "control" group was subjected to the hospital's standard practices. Parents were not allowed to accompany their children to the ward and said farewell to them in the admitting office. (The child was often dragged screaming from the office by nurses.) Not having the parents accompany the children to the wards, it was felt, helped reduce disruptive emotional scenes that might interfere with the routines in the wards. Visitation of parents was restricted for the same reasons. It seemed to make the children upset and this disrupted activities on the ward. No organized program of preventive or supportive emotional care of these patients or their families existed.

Striking (even terrifying) differences were found between the control and experimental groups. The children in the control group exhibited much more frequent, severe emotional reactions to hospitalization. These reactions persisted long after discharge.

Times have changed, fortunately, and whatever emotional scars parents have as a result of childhood hospitalization experiences, they need not be inflicted on their children. Almost all hospitals have programs that go beyond those suggested by the Children's Hospital's "radical" experimental program. Rooming-in arrangements are common, and parents are usually encouraged to take an active part in the care of a hospitalized child. Most hospitals have programs to familiarize children with the hospital prior to admission. None of these activities completely eliminates the emotional problems involved, but certainly it is a vastly improved situation from that of 35 years ago (Prugh et al. 1953, paraphrased).

Why did these changes take place? The development and widespread use of antibiotics certainly played a role. Evaluations such as the one described above also had an impact. In the last chapter we described the sources of change and the seemingly impersonal mechanics by which changes in organizational systems take place. In this chapter and the last one, we focus on the choices individuals within these systems can make concerning change. In this chapter we outline the alternative means, or tactics, individuals should consider for achieving change; in the final chapter we look at the alternative ends, or outcomes.

ALTERNATIVE ORIENTATIONS

How one deals with change depends on where one sits. Many individuals and groups view organizations as impersonal adversaries, while others see them as a means to an end. They want something from the organization, whether it is a better salary, better working conditions, or better care. As suggested in chapter 6, how much of these things they get depends on how much power or influence they have and the skill with which they use it.

During the 1960s, Lincoln Hospital, a municipal hospital in New York City, did relatively well in its attempts to influence the hospital corporation to provide it with a larger share of the budget. The combination of a takeover by the Young Lords, a radical Puerto Rican political group, and a job action that involved withholding Medicare and Medicaid reimbursement forms from the corporation emphasized the importance of Lincoln Hospital's needs in the minds of the corporation's management. The corporation has since given Lincoln Hospital increases that are substantially greater than those given other hospitals. Indeed, the corporation's formula for determining the budgets of its hospitals actually includes a "flak factor," providing additional money to institutions most likely to protest their budgets (Warner 1973).

Harlem Hospital, the other hospital to do relatively well in terms of increases in this budgeting process, also enjoyed an activist reputation. (A collective action by residents and members of the medical staff there once held up rush-hour traffic for several hours and gained immediate budgetary concessions.) Other municipal hospitals caught on, organizing their own radical medical action committees and indignant consumer representatives to highlight their needs and the callous indifference of the high-salaried, central Worth Street bureaucrats. Such competing attempts at influence pervade all health institutions and the system as a whole.

Unfortunately, as Tom Wolfe noted in his classic parody of the style, community efforts often lack the sustained pressure to assure results.

> Somehow it always seems to happen that way. Nobody ever follows it up. You can get everything together once, for the demonstration, for the confrontation, to go downtown and mau-mau, for the fun, for the big show, for the beano, for the main event, to see the people bury some gray cat's nuts and make him crawl and whine and sink in his own terrible grin. But nobody ever follows it up. You just sleep it off until somebody tells you there's going to be another big show.

And then later on you think about it and you say, "What really happened that day? Well, another flak catcher lost his manhood, that's what happened." Hmmmmmm . . . like maybe the bureaucracy isn't so dumb after all . . . All they did was sacrifice one flak catcher, and they've got hundreds, thousands . . . They've got replaceable parts. They threw this sacrifice to you, and you went away pleased with yourself. And even the Flak Catcher himself wasn't losing much. He wasn't losing his manhood. He gave that up a long time ago, the day he became a lifer . . . Just who is fucking over who . . . You did your number and he did his number, and they didn't even have to stop the music . . . The band played on . . . *Still*—did you see the *look* on his face? That sucker—" (Wolfe 1971, 118–19).

The efforts of persons who work within the health sector to influence health services organizations are far more focused and sustained. Since they view their task more as a long-term war than as a single battle, they are usually more effective. Obstetricians and surgeons, quick to take advantage of declining occupancy rates in many facilities, have extracted concessions from management. Because many facilities are financially dependent on their patronage, these physicians usually have only to scowl rather than resort to militant confrontations. Professional associations have been quite effective in shaping the reimbursement system and the licensing and regulation of health providers to the advantage of their members (Feldstein 1977). Nonprofessional workers have, similarly, succeeded in extracting some of what they want through collective bargaining agreements. As noted in chapter 6, this has resulted, at least in New York in the past, in Medicaid "passthroughs," or contracts, particularly in a gubernatorial election year.

Interest-group politics pervades the system. Those who are able to play well and have the resources and skills necessary to be effective will receive a disproportionate share of the rewards in terms of better pay, more autonomy, better care, and other privileges. Conflict becomes a tool for gaining such goals, rather than something that is disruptive and should be minimized. Discontent becomes a way of mobilizing the political power of a particular group. Much of this power may lie dormant most of the time; indeed, many participants may not even realize they have any power until they are sufficiently angered. Discontent may then create opportunities for the group—or it may endanger the group's ability to influence outcomes.

Organizations are more than just a conglomeration of groups and individuals competing in their own interests. Organizations are power holders. Their power was obtained presumably to serve collective purposes. From their perspective, the object is to manage, minimize, and control conflict so that common goals can be achieved more effectively, or at least so that the roof does not cave in when groups pursue their own interests. If the organization is to achieve its collective objectives, it must regulate conflict and minimize the disruptive effect of competitive struggles for influence. Commitment becomes the most important, difficult resource to obtain and maintain; discontent, alienation, apathy, the most serious problems. The flak catcher, as Wolfe suggests, performs a useful control function for the organization, allowing it to absorb a large amount of discontent at relatively little cost. Persons in public relations and, often, hospital administrators themselves (if they are so unfortunate as to be unable to avoid such a function) play the role of flak catcher.

People seeking influence and people seeking control both want change, but their goals are quite different. Those concerned with influence want something for themselves or for the group they represent; those concerned with control simply want to keep the whole organization from falling apart. They represent two sides of the same coin—and the same tactics, strategy, and alternative organizational models apply whether the concern is with influence or with control (Gamson 1968).

ALTERNATIVE TACTICS

When it comes to actually making a change, the choices tend to boil down to two: one can try to cram change down individual or collective throats, or one can try to win the hearts and minds of those involved.

Power struggles underlie many efforts to impose change on organizations. They operate where there is essentially a fixed-sum game—that is, where what one individual or group wins, the other individual or group loses. The attempt to change attitudes tends to exist in nonzero-sum games—that is, where both parties have something to gain, or at least one will not gain something at the expense of the other. For example, England has successfully reduced its suicide rate, while the United States has failed. Why? In England, the needed intervention did not require the government to take anything away from anyone, while in the United States it did. The most common means of suicide in England was domestic gas, whereas in the United States it was handguns. Laws lowering the carbon monoxide content of gas did not affect any interest group adversely, but laws restricting access to handguns did. As a result, the carbon monoxide content of domestic gas was reduced in England, but laws restricting access to handguns have failed to pass in the United States and the rate of suicide committed with handguns continues to rise.

Let us look at how similar dynamics work in hospitals.

Change in an Urban Teaching Hospital:
A Nonzero-Sum Game

This was a city hospital which had a close association with a medical school. Both hospital and school were venerable institutions with reputations for being among the best in their part of the continent. . . . The doctors were also aware that the medical field was advancing by strides and that to maintain status they would have to put forth effort to keep up and to achieve recognition for competence from their own professional associations. It might be said that the total environment was stimulating individuals to grow, while, in turn, these individuals, by growing, helped to stimulate each other, thus increasing the tempo of total change. There was a period of almost universal striving on the part of individuals and groups.

The administrators were in the forefront of all these developments, smoothing the way for them and struggling to keep abreast of change too. . . . They relished the struggle and soon became leaders in their own professional organizations, encouraging the pooling of knowledge and techniques among administrators from all over the nation. In other words, just as the doctors were becoming specialists, so were they. They kept pace.

What would have happened to them if they hadn't continued to grow? Would they have been able to coordinate effectively their increasingly alert and ambitious staff? As it was, the board, the administration, and the medical staff were growing and changing all at the same time and in so doing, kept and renewed the respect they held for one another. No one group could afford to shrug off the opinions of another, for all were of recognized competence in their own area.

It should by no means be assumed the human relations in this hospital were entirely comfortable. Probably there were just as many problems as in any other institution, but to the outsider it appeared that a feeling of accomplishment underlay the ebb and flow of daily events. People were too busy to fret much about changes in personal advantage from one week to the next. Each was hard at work, growing with the institution. There was a common pride in their individual progress and in belonging to an organization that was recognized by all as increasing in esteem both locally and nationally (Burling, Lentz, and Wilson 1956, 67–69).

Change in the Laboratory Department: A Zero-Sum Game

The assistant administrator of a 300-bed suburban hospital had just completed his analysis of the laboratory department and was pleased with his work. Careful adjustments in staffing to reflect day-of-the-week fluctuation in demand would produce some reduction in staffing, a substantial reduction in overtime pay, and a savings of about $300,000, or about 20 percent of the laboratory's labor costs. These savings could be achieved while at the same time reducing delays in reporting times. The pathologist, who was paid a percentage of the laboratory's gross, did not share the young administrator's pleasure. "What kind of silly nonsense is this? The patient's needs have to come first in any laboratory I'm involved in!" (That is, to hell with unit costs; maximize the volume and consequently my own income.) With a little luck, and some support at the board level, the administrator should be able to persevere (the balance of power produced by the changes in reimbursement and the ease of recruiting pathologists has shifted recently in the administrator's favor), but it will not be easy or bloodless (Griffith 1972; paraphrased).

Power Tactics

Power tactics make use of economic, political, and moral sanctions to create either the control or influence desired. Individuals or groups can be controlled by threats of demotion, salary cut, or loss of job and by threats of legal action. Institutions can be influenced by threats of strikes, boycotts, and sabotage.

Such tactics require an effective power base. Interest groups or bureaucrats that can supply power or place control of funding in determined hands can guarantee quick action. For example, racial integration of hospitals throughout the country in the 1960s was achieved far more quietly and expeditiously than integration of public schools. Why? Did people have different attitudes about sharing a hospital room with a member of a different race than they did about their children sharing a classroom? Probably not. However, the cash flow from federal Medicare and Medicaid programs, which added up to more than 50 percent of most hospitals' income, was something most facilities could not ignore. With local civil rights groups acting as watchdogs and consistent enforcement by federal officials, integration proceeded rapidly and with little of the belligerence that marred school integration. Although it is likely that more single-bed rooms were built than would otherwise have been built, this radical social transformation took place practically overnight.

Power tactics such as this, however, are truly effective only if certain conditions are met (Zaltman and Duncan 1977). First, such changes need not require individuals' commitment to the change, just their compliance. Nobody's attitude was changed overnight by the integration of hospitals. Second, such changes require the capability for enforcement. In the case of hospital integration, it was relatively easy to monitor enforcement, and the ultimate leverage of withholding Medicare and Medicaid funds was always available. Finally, there must be a reasonable expectation that there are individuals in the community who are favorably disposed toward the change. Local civil rights groups and an emerging national consensus supported the integration efforts; had neither existed, the efforts would probably have failed.

Attitude Change

The Rational Approach. Many situations involve nonzero sums, in which all parties would seem to benefit from the changes. Tactics aimed at changing attitudes seem to make more sense in such situations. There are two kinds of assumptions about people (paralleling the bureaucratic and participatory approaches suggested in chapter 4) that shape tactics for changing attitudes. One can assume that people are "rational," that is, that they are capable of analyzing data and agreeing on similar conclusions about the nature of the problem and appropriate actions. Evaluation researchers in the health area, as well as operations researchers and others involved in organizational research and development, usually make this assumption.

As in the case of the treatment of children in hospitals, one assumes that the results speak for themselves and that the appropriate changes will be almost automatic. One can facilitate this rational attitude toward change, as suggested in the previous chapter, by assuring a free flow of information through feedback on performance (Nadler 1977). Bringing more resources to bear on the identification of problems and the search for solutions will also speed such a process of change. Activities that bring different disciplines together to solve common problems have sometimes proved effective in facilitating change (Wieland and Bradford 1981). Outside consultants can provide key members of the organization with the additional information needed to facilitate the adoption of changes. Even the most obviously valuable, nonthreatening changes that develop from such rational-empirical analysis, however, often meet with disaster.

The Battle of the Intravenous Solutions

The hospital where I worked was an active member of the Chicago Hospital Council. At this time the Council was working on the idea of joint purchasing contracts for all 26 member hospitals. It was believed that considerable savings could be obtained on high-volume articles if one contract was negotiated through competitive bidding rather than 26 contracts. This proved to be true. For the one time in the history of the Council, it appeared that all 26 hospitals agreed on something. Member hospitals could receive significantly lower costs by purchasing items through the council contract rather than independently. The cost savings were so great that they overcame any feelings of loss of independence. The Council was together and they were strong. Competition for contracts among suppliers became fierce. The most hotly contested item was I.V. solutions. Baxter and Abbott Laboratories fought to the bitter end, with Baxter finally getting the contract by giving a price 80% *below catalog.*

Hospitals can generally be referred to as either "Baxter" or "Abbott" hospitals because they tend to buy their I.V.'s from one or the other company and never mix. We were an Abbott hospital which now required a change to become a Baxter. The solutions produced by each company could be assumed to be identical except for the trade names given to different types depending on the percent dextrose, glucose, etc. In the past I.V.'s had always been ordered by the purchasing agent (a registered pharmacist) and a memo was sent to each member of the medical staff informing them of new mixtures, mixture changes, etc., whenever appropriate. When the Council contract was signed, the medical staff was informed of the change and what it meant in terms of cost savings to the hospital and the patient. Although the change included new trade names for each solution, it was anticipated that this would not be a problem because three-fourths of the medical staff belonged to the staff of other nearby hospitals —all of which were Baxter hospitals. Thus they would no longer have to remember two different sets of trade names depending on which hospital they were in.

In spite of the overwhelming evidence that this change was for the better and that it was easier for the medical staff, the staff blocked the introduction of the Baxter solutions. It seems the Abbott salesman was calling the staff at night asking "Are you going to let administration tell you what type of I.V. to hang? Isn't this a medical question? Who is in control here anyway? It finally ended when Abbott agreed to meet Baxter's price. We remained an Abbott hospital and the council suffered a blow because we had to withdraw from the joint contract (Ries 1974, 3–6).

The ultimate in rational change, computerized information systems have had more than their fair share of difficulties in implementation in health facilities. One study suggests that about 45 percent of short-term hospitals that have implemented such systems have experienced staff "interference" (Dowling 1980). That interference has come in the form of refusing to cooperate, spreading dissatisfaction with the system, putting off learning about the system and making "errors," and sabotaging the data on the system. One medical technician, for example, deliberately misplaced leads and used insufficient electrolytic cream for proper contact on persons undergoing EKGs, thereby convincing his superiors that there was a serious malfunction of the equipment. Reassigning the technician to other duties finally solved the problem. A clerk in a clinical laboratory succeeded in bringing the implementation of a new system to a standstill. Physicians complained about the inaccuracy of the information produced: normal values for tests were incorrect, and many of the "newborn" patients in the data system had wives and children. The errors ended only after the clerk was threatened with dismissal if the problems, which the clerk denied having any role in, didn't stop.

All of this is not to belittle the value of fact gathering, experimentation, and analysis. Transforming alternatives into numerical outcomes makes the consequences visible. It also makes the values underlying certain decisions, as well as the power that shapes them, all too clear. Such visibility can lessen the impact of raw power on decision making. This helps create new criteria upon which those decisions can be based, criteria more open to debate and criticism.

The Psychological Approach. The right setting, the right data, the right analysis, and the right options are rarely enough to induce change. Strategies for changing attitudes usually require more than simply the dissemination of information to be effective. (If this were the case, rates of change would be similar in different organizational settings, and adoption of new technologies or ideas among individuals would occur at random.) Individuals have certain psychological needs that must be met, and these needs are both impediments to and potential allies in obtaining change.

Social psychologists have devoted a good deal of effort to the study of attitude change. Varela (1971) has presented some useful, although unnerving, ways of applying the results to the manipulation of real people. Some of the key factors to keep in mind in designing persuasions are summarized here.*

Use Successive Approximation: Individuals' attitudes about something like a new program in a hospital will vary. They may feel very positive about certain aspects of it and strongly negative about other aspects. For example, physicians tend to feel quite positive about the greater technical capabilities of a prepaid group practice and the environment surrounding it, which seems more conducive to acquiring new skills and keeping up to date, but they feel quite negative about other aspects of salaried practice, such as income restrictions and the potential for abuse of their services by patients (McElrath 1961). These attitudes can be arrayed along a continuum, from those of physicians who strongly accept the idea to those of physicians who strongly object to it (presumably the attitude one wishes to change). It seems that the most effective strategy is to proceed by "successive approximations," trying to change first the attitude of the physician who only mildly disagrees with the idea. This approach tends to make the individual feel less negative toward other attitudes and closer to the attitude one is trying to get the person to adopt. That is, "the latitude of rejection changes and the person's position on the issue is less extreme" (Varela 1971, 87). As part of an overall persuasion effort, successive approximation seems to promise greater chances of success than immediate confrontation of the individual who is most strongly opposed.

Avoid Reactance: In general, effective persuasion seems to work best when a person is unaware of attempts to influence him or her. The greater and more obvious the pressures placed on individuals, the more likely they are to resist. Positions may harden, and individuals may even move in the opposite direction. (This possibility is used to good advantage by Varela in the persuasion design that follows.) Even if the pressure is sufficiently great to cause the person to make certain limited concessions, he or she is likely to refuse to budge on subsequent occasions. The following case illustrates how *successive approximation* and *reactance* can be used to achieve a desired persuasion.

---

*This section relies heavily on Varela (1971, 83–142). Our own account is abbreviated and oversimplified, therefore we refer the interested reader to Varela's book and the more basic research references he supplies.

Figure 8.1   Design of a Persuasion

Joe's
Initial Position – ▶Agreement

I				II	III	IV	V	VI

Key
Statement

Joe's Initial
Attitude*

I:	I love my family very much	+5
II:	I spend very little time with my family	−1
III:	My health is much worse now than when I was a young man	−2
IV:	I have not provided for my family's future	−3
V:	At my age, health problems arise which if left untended may turn into something serious but which can be prevented by early detection	−4
VI:	I should go now and get a medical checkup	−5

*Attitudes range from +5 (strongly agree) to −5 (strongly disagree).

Persuasion by Successive Approximation, Using Reactance

How do you persuade someone to get a medical checkup you suspect he needs? Figure 8.1 summarizes the attitudes of this hard-driven ulcer-prone executive and devoted family man. With this road map of his attitudes, you know where you have to move him, and you do it by engaging him in a dialogue (albeit abbreviated) something like this:

X: You know, Joe, I don't think you really care much about your family. (This creates reactance, causing Joe to strongly affirm statement I and reduce his negative reaction to statement II.)

Joe: Why would you say such a thing?

X: Well, maybe I'm wrong, but in what ways do you show it?

Joe: I do everything I can to look after them and make sure the kids get the best education possible. I work hard for them.

X: Yeah, I guess I was wrong, you do spend a lot of time with your family. (Reactance will now push an annoyed Joe to disagree with statement II.)

Joe: No, not half the time I'd like to, work pressures being what they are. (Reactance enabled him to change his attitude; statement II is now at +1, rather than −1.)

X: That's too bad, but you're lucky you're still in as good health as when you were starting out so you can deal with the long hours and pressure. (Reactance again.)

Joe: Well, I think I'm pretty healthy, but it can't compare to when I was much younger.

X: Well, even if your health isn't as good, and working as hard as you say you do it might continue to decline, I'm sure you've made financial arrangements for your family should something happen to you.

Joe: No, I can't really say that I have. We haven't been able to save much, and I haven't much in the way of disability insurance should I become ill. (Joe now moves to the right of statement IV; he would now rate the statement +1, a big jump forced by the dissonance between his strongly felt concerns about his family and his lack of attention to these matters.)

X: Well, nothing happens to people in our age group. You're safe.

Joe: But Bill had a serious problem with ulcers; he should have taken care of it much sooner.

X: What should he have done?

Joe: Should have seen a doctor. I guess we're all pretty foolish on that score. Mary's been after me for some time to see a doctor. (Joe recognized the analogy to his own case and has now moved to +1 on statement VI. This is, of course, a very abbreviated version of a persuasion that should last at least half an hour, moving the individual through very gradual commitments and allowing time for the dissonance between attitudes to lessen. Also, attitude change must be translated into action.)

X: That's not a bad idea, but what are you going to do about it?

Joe: I'm not sure who to go to. It's been a long time since I've been to a doctor.

X: Why don't you give your wife a call? She knows the name of Bill's physician, but you'd better tell her what it's about. (By getting Joe heavily committed to following through, the persuader hopes to avoid the problem of post-decision regret. He's got Joe nailed down) (Varela 1971, 89–93; paraphrased).

Use of Analogy: Using an example that is unrelated to the attitude problem at hand but that elicits from the individual a personal commitment to the logic involved can prove quite useful. Such an unrelated discussion has the advantage of not touching on sensitive vested interests and avoiding previously induced reactance. It has been shown that individuals seem to need to perceive themselves as consistent. If an individual buys the logic in an unrelated context and then sees its inconsistency with the argument he is using in the current context, he will experience a certain amount of tension, or dissonance. This dissonance can only be relieved by some change in his previously held position. The basic logic underlying some people's resistance to seeing a doctor, for example, is as follows:

1. People who are not ill should not consult doctors.
2. I am not ill.
3. Therefore I should not consult a doctor (Varela 1971, 94).

One might begin by trying to change the first rather than the third premise, for which an individual has probably built up a good deal of reactance to change. If one is able to change the initial premise, then the individual is likely to experience a certain amount of dissonance. Change can be brought about by describing a concrete, analogous case that the individual is familiar with, such as the parallel that was drawn between Joe's and Bill's situations in the example earlier.

In persuading someone to accept new programs or technologies within an institution, it may be useful to lead the individual to express approval of similar types of programs in other settings. For example, convincing an individual of the usefulness of operations research methods in the space program could make persuading him of their usefulness in solving complex problems within his own institution flow more smoothly.

Apply Social Pressure: Groups tend to exert a great deal of pressure toward conformity. Early experiments in social psychology demonstrated that, if naive subjects are placed in a group of confederates who agree to incorrectly judge the length of a line, more than one-third of the subjects will conform to those judgments, and many of the remainder will experience a good deal of tension and confusion (Asch 1952). Similar effects of group pressure have been obtained using attitude statements (Crutchfield 1955). In order for the conformity effect to be present, it seems that at least four persons acting in concert are needed; greater majorities do little to improve the effect. Peer pressure is undoubtedly used intuitively by adept administrators to manipulate committee members and hospital board members.

The New Wing

The hospital board has been called together to decide between two alternative designs for a new wing. The administrator prefers the modern, glass structure. The most influential board member, however, prefers the more conservative design, which looks more like the bank he represents. The administrator seats the board members in such a way that they cannot see each others' faces but the administrator has a clear view of each of them. He will then proceed with a discussion of the options, complete with flip charts and slides. He makes his pitch for the glass facility and scans his audience for signs of approval and disapproval. The bank representative frowns, but another member leans forward with interest and nods his head slightly. The administrator turns to this board member and asks his opinion of the option. The board member indicates that he likes it, and the administrator asks him why. (This helps obtain full commitment from the individual and also allows the administrator to scan the group for signs of approval from the other members.) Some of the things the board member says are likely to trigger signs of approval from other members, and the administrator seeks their opinion. The most influential, resisting member will, of course, be left until last. By this time he should be feeling sufficient pressure to revise his opinions about the modernistic structure somewhat. (More rigid, authoritarian individuals tend to have a low tolerance for ambiguity and seem to be more susceptible to such pressures.) The seating arrangements have prevented the more ingratiating members of the board from giving initial support to the banker. The administrator will get his glass edifice.

In general, persuasion tactics need to take into account the dynamics of groups. Attempts to influence people tend to be filtered, interpreted, and evaluated by individual "opinion leaders" within groups. These opinion leaders are heavily relied on by other members of the group in forming their own opinions.

The power of a group over the attitudes and behaviors of its members, however, is contingent on a number of factors. In order for the group to be influential, the individual must feel a sense of belonging to it. The more attractive the group is to the individual, the greater its influence over him. The most effective tactics for group change take advantage of these influences. At the very least, information concerning the need for a particular change needs to be mulled over and discussed within the group rather than seeming to be imposed from the outside. If a shared perception that a particular change is needed can possibly be developed within a group, then all is likely to flow smoothly. Identifying and dealing with the opinion leaders of such groups can facilitate this process. The I.V. solution case presented earlier would probably have been relatively easy to push through if an intelligent attempt had been made to cope with some of these principles of group dynamics within the medical staff.

Gain Commitment Through Compliance with Small Requests: Further commitments can often be gained from individuals by first obtaining small, seemingly reasonable requests. This strategy is similar to that of successive approximation described previously. In one experiment, housewives were contacted by telephone and told that a market research survey was being taken; they were asked to answer a few questions about the products they were using. Later, the housewives were contacted again and asked to allow a team of male researchers to enter and make a detailed search of their homes, identifying all the products they used. Over half of those who had complied with the first request agreed to the second, whereas only 22 percent of those who had not complied with the first request agreed to the second (Freedman and Fraser 1966).

The area of health care would seem to offer many opportunities for applying a similar strategy. For example, a public interest group that wishes to publish a consumer's guide to physicians in a given community should not begin by trying to develop a complete dossier on each physician. The group might first limit itself to requesting permission to publish physicians' telephone numbers and information that is available in the American Medical Association directory for the group's own use. After this initial commitment was obtained, the group might be able to add in subsequent years more sensitive information, such as fees for various procedures, hospital privileges, willingness to prescribe contraceptives to sexually active minors, and so forth, with less likelihood of encountering violent resistance from the local medical society.

Use Distraction to Facilitate Persuasion: Experiments in social psychology have shown that persuasion is likely to be most effective when the subject is not forewarned and there are sufficient distractions to prevent his marshalling a counterargument. Thus, effective persuasion should, at the very least, start with some kind of distraction. This has apparently always been a part of the bag of tricks of salesmen and con artists. Dale Carnegie students are instructed to begin each sales pitch with an amusing personal story. This helps distract the listener from the speaker's purpose and allows him to see the speaker in more friendly terms rather than as a potential adversary. When skillfully executed, this technique is virtually foolproof—except when the persuader is confronted with another hardened graduate of the Dale Carnegie school (Kovner 1974).

> *Salesman:* On my way to the hospital this morning I happened to pass a little old man who was . . .
>
> *Administrator:* (slamming his fist on the table in rage) Don't give me any of that Dale Carnegie bullshit!
>
> *Salesman:* (cringing slightly, but forcing a determined, beneficent grin and desperately trying to formulate a Dale Carnegie contingency plan) Now, Bob . . .

Most distractions need not be elaborate; they simply involve engaging the victim in an unrelated conversation or activity. A game of golf is perhaps the most traditional ruse used in administrative and medical circles. Because of this, it is probably no longer particularly effective, and the creative persuader would do well to look for other kinds of distractions.

Use Food: Some evidence suggests that offering food facilitates persuasion (Janis, Kaye, and Kirshner 1965). Another study notes that free food has a fairly limited effect, because it induces compliance only while it is being consumed (Dabbs and Janis 1965). Nevertheless, food seems to be a widespread component of persuasion in the area of health care. It is an integral part of the professional socialization process: drug companies frequently treat medical students, interns, and residents to steak dinners and weekend vacations near company headquarters during so-called company tours. Such activities are continued after physicians are in private practice, with detail men usually inviting them to lunch. A hospital bed and casket company has traditionally provided weekend hospitality to entire classes of hospital administration students. The company plane flies them to a plush country club retreat, and a tour of the bed and casket factories is sandwiched in between a heavy schedule of eating and drinking. Health care administrators often follow similar tactics in the care and feeding of their boards. Beginning meetings with a heavy luncheon tends to assure a reasonably compliant, if not somnambulant, board.

Take Advantage of Curiosity: Curiosity has not only killed the cat, it has also succeeded in unloading a lot of new technology on physicians and hospitals. Some of this equipment is useful, but much of it is worthless. Both animals and human beings are attracted and motivated to explore the new and unfamiliar. Such motivations have long been taken advantage of by astute salesmen.

Salesman: Let's see, I've got some of the more standard stuff in the bottom of this case. (The salesman carefully lifts a small shiny gadget and places it ever so slowly on the side of the desk and then returns to rummage in the bottom of his case.)

Pathologist: Hey, what's that thing?

Salesman: Oh, that's the new _____. I don't think you'd have any interest in it, only the big teaching hospitals in the city are using it.

Pathologist: Oh yeah, why not?

Salesman: Oh, I doubt you do many of those kinds of tests in a hospital like this.

Pathologist: That's not true! We do some of those.

Salesman: Well, it's pretty expensive and Anderson (the administrator) would probably put up a big fuss about purchasing it.

Pathologist: That jackass! What the hell does he know? I'll make the medical decisions in this department. Show me how it works!

Skillful use of curiosity combined with reactance that takes advantage both of sensitive professional pride and traditional medical-administrative antagonisms has enabled the salesman to actually maneuver the pathologist into persuading *him* that the hospital needs the gadget. If the salesman had tried to sell the item directly, the pathologist would probably have told him that it was too damned expensive and that the hospital would have little use for it. Instead, the hospital is likely to buy a new gadget that will spend most of its time gathering dust.

There are, of course, more socially useful purposes to which such persuasive behavior can be put. Administrators may find it more useful to have medical staff abuses or inequities of care "discovered" by other medical staff members in a routine presentation of hospital operations than to point them out themselves. (This assumes, of course, that the presentation is designed in such a way that the aberrations will not go unnoticed.)

Such techniques are based on certain pernicious assumptions about people: that they are incapable of making rational decisions and that they need to be manipulated by those persons who know best. It is a difficult set of ethical dilemmas to untangle, yet each individual must confront and resolve them to the best of his or her ability. In attempting to reach some resolution, three points should be considered:

1. These techniques are likely to be used by the relatively power-less. The powerful, authoritarian official has neither the need nor the inclination to engage in such subtleties.

2. The persons most likely to abuse these techniques already know, at least intuitively, how to use them. No one is unleash-ing a new weapon on the naive, unsuspecting health care sys-tem. Persons who are less likely to abuse the techniques need to know about them in order to become resistant to them.

3. Finally, there are clear limits to how far these techniques can be abused. If the actions taken are clearly detrimental to the indi-viduals persuaded, the whole thing is likely to blow up in the persuader's face. People will eventually realize that they have been conned. Further persuasions will be more difficult and eventually impossible. For such tactics to be effective in the long run, an atmosphere of trust, openness, and mutual respect must be maintained.

Combining Attitude Change and Power Tactics

Attitude change and power tactics represent two distinct traditions of analysis in social science. The power approach has been advanced by game theorists and students of diplomacy and revolutions. They have attempted to describe the development of a power base and the stra-tegic manipulation of that power to gain objectives. Social scientists representing attitude change have tended to advocate trust, openness, and mutual respect. The obvious tension between the proponents of these two strategies has generally been dealt with by either ignoring it or deprecating the other point of view. These conflicts and tensions, how-ever, cannot be ignored by anyone involved in change. Most situations are not clearly either a zero-sum or nonzero-sum game—they require a mixture of tactics.

There are some inherent problems in pursuing both of these tac-tics simultaneously. Attitude change tactics require the creation of an atmosphere of mutual trust and openness that enables individuals to al-ter previously held positions without a sense of failure or defeat. Power tactics require tighter, less open, more calculating behavior. The two are obviously difficult to mix (Walton 1969).

Overstating Objectives versus Deemphasizing Differences. Exagger-ating the differences between oneself and the individuals or groups one wants to influence or control may enable one to push them in the direc-tion one wants them to go. It is a standard tactic of both labor and management negotiators in collective bargaining, with both sides secretly prepared to settle for less than they are demanding. Such tactics run the risk of creating reactance, however, of convincing the other side that the differences are even greater than anticipated, that the gulf between the groups is too great, and that any basis for reconciliation is impossible. The result can be the creation of armed camps within an organization and sporadic warfare, sapping the energy of the organization and reducing avenues for influence and control.

Power to Coerce versus Trust. Emphasis on an individual's power to either enforce regulations within an institution or disrupt operations can be useful in obtaining control or concessions in the short run. Yet the kind of trust essential for long-term control or influence is unlikely to develop from such tactics. Trust is built by emphasizing both the importance of the group one is attempting to change and one's dependence on it, rather than by coercing the group. An administrator can, as in the previous case, impose standards on the staff in terms of legal requirements, but he is perhaps better off if, by emphasizing the hospital's dependence on the conduct of the doctors, he can get them to start thinking about the long-term survival of the institution rather than individual privileges.

Ambiguity versus Predictability of Information. Power tactics call for a high degree of ambiguity. The other side must not know precisely how far you are prepared to go.

> A handful of women, all expectant mothers, formed an organization and began trying to persuade the local hospital to allow husbands in the delivery room. The majority of the obstetricians were adamantly opposed, although the women were armed with evidence of the safety of such procedures in other hospitals. The women and their husbands deluged the local paper with letters to the editor, hounded the administrator and the various obstetricians, and, most important, publicized the fact that several women (the actual number was never specified) were traveling to a hospital outside the community to have their babies delivered in a hospital that permitted their husbands in the delivery room. They successfully created the illusion of a mass movement. The threat of a mass exodus was enough to bring the obstetricians around. A closer look at the potential for such an exodus would have revealed that at most it would involve only about a half-dozen deliveries a year. Real attitude change did not take

place. Such a change would have required much more open, less calculating communication between the two groups, which was not possible in this initial phase.

Threat versus Conciliation. Similarly, the balance between threats and conciliation must be carefully weighed. The recent development of business coalitions for health and their activities in support of controlling health care costs while maintaining adequate services for their employees demonstrate that businesses, patients, health professionals, and facilities can modify traditional conflict-of-interest behavior in order to work toward a common solution to critical problems. Relations among consumers, providers, institutions, third-party payers, government, and business have progressed through stormy and confused stages. Now some of these groups seem to be beginning an era of cooperative efforts to find new solutions to threatening dilemmas.

Impact of Hostility versus Catharsis. In terms of power tactics, hostility requires careful, calculated management that is designed to create the optimum impact on the adversary. Attitude change tactics require a less calculated venting of feelings that enables one to reevaluate his or her feelings with a minimum impact on others. For example, collective bargaining situations require carefully controlled hostility. While people need to represent their positions forcefully, they still have to work closely together afterwards. Sometimes people can forget when to turn hostility off.

> A bitter strike was over. The administration had been successful in preventing what it felt were highly inflationary wage demands by the nursing staff with some limited concessions. To celebrate the end of the strike, an open bar, caviar, and champagne party was sponsored by the administrator for the nursing staff and supervisors who had not honored the picket lines. The returning strikers were excluded. The next day, the hospital board, which had strongly backed the administrator in his negotiations with the nurses' union, asked for the administrator's resignation.

Coalition versus Inclusion. A final dilemma involving these two alternative tactics is how one goes about developing alliances. Power tactics would dictate building alliances with other groups *against* the group whose change is desired, while attitude change tactics would dictate including the group within whatever structure evolves, in hopes of changing members' attitudes through increased communication. Local coalitions have generally attempted to adopt the latter strategy, including various consumer groups within the same structure. Depending on one's perspective, this has led either to the total stagnation and emasculation of the health planning concept or to slow, imperceptible changes in attitude among the various consumer groups, changes that will eventually result in more effective planning of health care within a region.

Mixing Tactics

When using both tactics, as one must in many situations, one needs to weigh the benefits of a power tactic against the effect it will have on attitude change tactics. Gratuitous insults and provocative behavior that add little to a power strategy but increase the hostility of the persons whose attitudes must eventually be changed are obviously to be avoided. The nonviolent strategy of the early civil rights and peace movements attempted to integrate these tactics. It was not particularly successful, since the distinctions between nonviolent and violent behavior were generally meaningful only to those involved—and not to those in opposition to these causes. Similarly, obsequious, ingratiating behavior that adds nothing to attitude change objectives and that does not help in building a power strategy should be avoided.

Combining the two tactics can be quite effective if it is done skillfully. One can alternate them, first blowing hot and then cold. Both sides of the East-West conflict seem to have used such a freeze-thaw approach in attempting to gain concessions from each other. Union organizing efforts often combine these strategies, following militant demonstrations with a negotiation phase.

The tactics can be combined by having different persons or subgroups pursuing them separately. Violent confrontations by some of the groups' leaders can be combined simultaneously with appeals from other members for "understanding." Such a strategy is more effective for loosely bound social movements than for organizations in which one or the other leader would lose credibility.

Power tactics will almost inevitably prevail in situations where the balance of power is unequal. They may take a velvet-glove approach, but they will nonetheless be the primary determinants of change. For persons who lack influence, confrontation and power tactics are usually the only tactics available. Once such tactics are incorporated into the decision-making structure of an institution, however, attitude change tactics are the most effective, realistic way of achieving change. In short, in order to be an effective agent for change, one must develop the skills associated with both power and attitude change tactics and become sophisticated in mixing them.

STARTING POINTS:
INDIVIDUAL, ORGANIZATION, OR SYSTEM?

Where does one start in any effort to produce change? Does one first try to change individuals, organizations, or the environment within which they operate? It depends on whether one's perspective is that of influence or control and on how important one believes the needed changes are. If one is concerned about control, one will focus on changing individual behavior, either through selective recruitment or through offering the right rewards and motivation. If one is concerned about influence, one will be more concerned with changing organizational structure, or the system as a whole. Minor changes can be solved by tinkering at the individual level, while substantive changes require a radical restructuring of the entire system. Wherever one starts, however, changes at other levels will eventually be required.

Many programs designed to improve the climate within an organization by improving the attitudes of participants fail to take into account the need for concomitant structural change. What seems to be safe tinkering can backfire.

Employee of the Month

The personnel department of a large, prestigious teaching hospital was concerned about the morale of the nonprofessional employees. It hit on the idea of having these people vote for an individual who would be Employee of the Month. The winner was to receive a small cash award, and a large photograph of him or her was to be prominently displayed in the plush lobby of the hospital. The maintenance department employees, as well as some members of other departments, immediately saw the potential for humor in this and began discussing among themselves who had the potential for being the ugliest "playmate of the month." One candidate stood well above all the other contenders. He was referred to as "the troll." He was grotesquely physically deformed and slightly feeble-minded. He had a tiny receding chin and a beetle brow cast in a perpetual scowl. He became the overwhelming choice, receiving five times as many votes as the runner-up, an obese woman in the dietary department. His morose prominence decorated the hospital's well-appointed lobby for the next month, followed by others almost equally as well endowed. It took the personnel department four months to catch on. The winners caught on much sooner.

Often organizations can create structures that support and stimulate change. For example, quality circles are small groups of employees from the same areas of an organization working on problems to improve productivity and quality. Organizations have also found it useful to designate specific individuals as idea generators, sponsors, or orchestrators (Galbraith 1982). Creating such roles helps in identifying needed changes and carrying them through to implementation. Other types of integrating mechanisms, such as task forces and matrix structures (in which individuals from various specialty areas make decisions about a particular market they serve), can facilitate change (Mintzberg 1979, Kanter 1983).

Much change in the health sector, however, as we suggested in chapter 7, begins with changes in the system, or environment. These changes may involve shifts in payment, regulation, or market pressures, to which health service organizations and individuals must respond. Such systemwide changes are the province of social reformers, lobbyists for special-interest groups, and, increasingly often, administrators themselves.

The advocacy nature of systemwide efforts at change tends to simplify complexities and to present reform as a panacea. No matter how conceptually sound, however, systemwide changes cannot succeed without concomitant structural and individual changes. The shift to a prospective payment system, for example, has required concomitant shifts in the structure of health service organizations and in the way individuals within them function, shifts that are just beginning to be worked through. The final chapter suggests some alternative outcomes that might be achieved through such changes.

9

Endpoints

Voices

"It's horrible to die being pushed around like that. I know I don't want that for myself" (Alice Cramer's son).

"It's an exciting game. I can get all wrapped up in the wheeling and dealing, spinning off for-profit subsidiaries and developing joint ventures, and doing real corporate strategic planning without a lot of the old sacred cow prohibitions. Every once in a while, though, I stop and think, Wait a minute! Is this really why I went into this field? What does all this have to do with health care? Some of it just doesn't sit that well in my stomach" (CEO Fleet Foot Hospital).

"Doctors coin money when they do procedures—family practice doesn't have any procedures. A urologist has cystoscopies, a gastroenterologist has gastroscopies, a dermatologist has biopsies. They can do three or four of those and make five or six hundred dollars in a single day. We get nothing for the use of our time to understand the lives of our patients. Technology is rewarded in medicine, it seems to me, and not thinking" (a family practitioner in Maine, in McPhee 1984, 57).

"The ideas of economists and political philosophers both when they are right and when they are wrong are more powerful than is commonly understood. Indeed, the world is ruled by little else. Practical men, who believe themselves to be quite exempt from any intellectual influences, are usually the slave of some defunct economist. Madmen in authority, who hear voices in the air, are distilling their frenzy from some academic scribbler a few years back. I am sure that the power of vested interests is vastly exaggerated compared to the gradual encroachment of ideas" (Keynes 1936, 383).

"Would you tell me, please, which way I ought to go from here?"

"That depends a good deal on where you want to get to," said the Cat.

"I don't much care where . . ." said Alice.

"Then it doesn't matter which way you go," said the Cat.

". . . so long as I get somewhere," Alice added as an explanation.

"Oh you're sure to do that," said the Cat, "if you only walk long enough."

Alice felt that this could not be denied, so she tried another question. "What sort of people live about here?"

"In THAT direction," the Cat said, waving his paw around, "lives a Hatter; and in THAT direction," waving his other paw, "lives a March Hare. Visit either you like; they're both mad."

"But I don't want to go among mad people," Alice remarked.

"Oh, you can't help that," said the Cat, "we're all mad here. I'm mad. You're mad."

"How do you know I'm mad?" said Alice.

"You must be," said the Cat, "or you wouldn't have come here" (Carroll 1946, 62–63).

Alice Cramer's son, Fleet Foot's CEO, and the family practitioner in Maine all share a similar discomfort. Whatever ideas they have, or have incorporated in some circuitous way from those "academic scribblers," about how things should work do not fit their experience. We have tried to provide in this book better directions than the Cheshire Cat gave Alice. At the very least, one should be able to recognize the Alice-in-Wonderland madness of many of the more simplistic solutions that are currently being offered.

Our review of the development of the health sector in chapter 1 emphasized the cyclical concerns that have guided its evolution and dramatic expansion. Health care has been defined at different times as predominantly an economic good, a professional service, and a social relationship. The persistence of these conflicting definitions has made it impossible, and probably will continue to make it impossible, to treat health care simply as another economic good that should be subjected to the same free play of market forces as any other good or to treat it as something that should be completely insulated from market forces.

The description of the mechanics of the system, in chapter 2, should make one wary of the unintended consequences of simply treating the symptoms of a particular element of that complex system. Different gateways shape demand, supply, and production of services within the system, but they cannot be isolated from each other. A capitation arrangement, a fixed-rate reimbursement by admission, and so on all have ripple effects on other providers, patterns of utilization, and, ultimately, the health of the population, whether care is defined as an economic good, a professional service, or a social relationship.

Assessment of existing performance in terms of access, cost, efficiency, effectiveness, and equity, as presented in chapter 3, should give us some sense of humility about the ease with which any outcome can be changed. Improvements in one of these performance criteria are usually obtained at the expense of another. Improved access, for example, produces increased cost and reduced efficiency, while more effective control of costs usually reduces accessibility and equity.

The relationship between organizations and their environments described in chapter 4 underscores two basic organizational problems that hinder satisfactory performance.

First, there are conflicting assumptions about how health care should be organized. The conflicting perceptions and values underlying them are part of the environment from which organizations develop. Three models of organization, bureaucratic, professional, and participatory, compete for dominance within the health care structure. The tensions produced by these conflicting models are part of the day-to-day strain experienced in almost every health service organization.

Second, organizations respond to environmental pressures in such a way as to minimize disruption of existing operations. In most cases this will limit the organization's ability to respond to changes in the environment, thus reducing the overall performance of the system.

Similar factors limit the ability and willingness of individuals to respond to the needs of an organization, as described in chapter 5. Bureaucratic, professional, and participatory models of organization have analogues in the three major orientations of transactional analysis (parent, adult, and child). Individuals experience stress in responding to changes in their environment and attempt to insulate themselves from rapid change.

Individuals work together and create organizations only when all parties benefit from the exchange. What an individual or an organization can command for such participation depends on its power, as suggested in chapter 6. On the individual level, such power is related to position, expert knowledge, personal charisma, and the leverage associated with an individual's ability to leave an organization if it fails to be responsive to his concerns. Individuals also have power in relationship to the groups to which they belong. On the organizational level, power is associated with size, ownership, centralization of control, and specialization. These attributes tend to be associated with the bureaucratic model and tend to explain the drift toward it. On the system level, power includes whatever is not absorbed by individuals and organizations, and it determines the degree to which the system can control or become the captive of the organizations that make it up.

In chapter 7 we describe how changes in organizational structures and systems come about. Changes may represent planned, controlled responses of an organization—what is referred to as a strategic planning or marketing approach to the environment—or the unplanned influence of political constituencies within the organization or its environment.

Finally, in chapter 8 we discuss tactics for speeding up or slowing down such processes of change. The effects of influence versus control are explored, as well as attitude change versus power tactics. The close relationship between structure and outcomes was again emphasized, since part of any individual or group strategy involves shaping the playing field to its own advantage.

OPTIONS IN STRUCTURING HEALTH CARE

What remains is for us to sketch in more detail the potential consequences of all of these pressures in the form of alternative outcomes for the system as a whole. One can then support whichever scenario is more compatible with one's own values, career, interests, or preferences as a consumer of its services. No matter which scenario one chooses, however, a prolonged and difficult struggle will ensue.

We cannot deal with all the possible structural permutations of an organizational system as complex as the health sector. Instead, we will need to sort through the different possibilities, discarding some as irrelevant in the light of historical developments and current political realities and combining others under fairly simplistic headings. The objective is to clarify the kinds of choices we confront. To do so, we must create ideal types of those choices, recognizing that the organizational structures we actually deal with do not fit any of them.

Throughout this book we have suggested three alternative organizational models—the bureaucratic, professional, and participatory—as ways of sorting out these choices. These models imply particular styles and structures that have implications for (1) relationships between provider and patient (the micro level), (2) how work is organized in health settings (the intermediate level), and (3) how the system as a whole is controlled (the macro level). At each of these levels the models suggest alternatives for such basic structural characteristics as (1) size, (2) degree of centralization, and (3) specialization. Adopting a bureaucratic model implies the selection of a relatively larger operation, a greater degree of centralization of control, and a greater degree of specialization. The participatory model implies a smaller operation, a greater degree of decentralized control, and limited specialization.

Ownership, whether it is private, public, or voluntary, is not as tightly tied to organizational form. Small-scale entrepreneurial ventures by private firms, for example, can fit the participatory model, and large public-payment schemes such as the Health Care Financing Administration fit the bureaucratic model. Nevertheless, the basic trend has been toward larger operations, greater specialization, and greater centralization of control; ownership has changed from predominantly public to predominantly private.

Consequently, in this chapter we look at models that illustrate these trends—that is, at each of the three organizational forms (professional, bureaucratic, and participatory) on each of the three system levels (micro, intermediate, and macro). In order to illustrate the structural implications at each level, we take a widely advocated "solution" and show how it might be adapted to fit into each of these different types of organizational structures. Each of the popular solutions, as we have hinted earlier, has the chameleon's ability to change colors to match its surroundings. The appeal of these solutions is precisely their ambiguity. They create the illusion of value-free, nonzero-sum, scientific solutions, in which conflicting values and special interests play no role. While this may enhance their organizational and political acceptability, the truth is that they are not really solutions at all. They are an arena in which solutions (or ways of organizing activities) that can be responsive to quite different values and interests are worked out.

We first look at the choice that is least disruptive of the status quo —the professional structure on the micro level. We then move to the bureaucratic and participatory options at this level, and finally to the professional, bureaucratic, and participatory options on the intermediate and macro levels. We move from choices that involve only minor operational tinkering to choices that involve radical changes in both organizational goals and organizational structures. Yet any major transformation, as we suggested in chapter 8, must include—indeed, often begin with—such minor operational tinkering. Expanded searches take place not just because of failure, but also because of success.

Alternatives on the Micro Level

One solution to the dilemmas of access, cost, efficiency, and effectiveness that has been advocated is the use of new health practitioners. Studies have suggested that much of a physician's practice time is wasted, in the sense that it is being spent on activities that could have been dealt with adequately by less costly, more narrowly trained personnel. Such individuals can (1) enhance access by providing a more plentiful supply of practitioners, particularly in underserved areas; (2) reduce cost by substituting their labor for more costly physician labor; (3) increase efficiency by improving overall productivity, as measured by cost per unit of service; and (4) increase effectiveness by placing a greater emphasis on prevention, health education, and early detection and treatment. Let us look at the organizational frameworks in which they might be placed.

Bureaucratic Structure. Both physician assistants and nurse practitioners have been used in large office practices and clinics to perform specialized, discrete tasks in the processing of patients. Veterans Administration facilities, large hospital-based clinics, and HMOs have been more aggressive in changing the structure of their outpatient practices to effectively utilize physician extenders. Their willingness stems in part from their acceptance of more bureaucratic modes of organization, but it also results from their not having to face the same third-party restrictions in the use of such practitioners that noninstitutional fee-for-service practitioners do.

One structure developed by a large HMO shows how bureaucratic rationality might be used to break the work performed in an outpatient setting down into specialized tasks, thereby assuring more limited reliance on physicians while increasing access to services (figure 9.1). In an initial evaluation of the system, it was found that only 26.8 percent of patient visits required physician contact (a number corresponding to the findings of other studies of the overlap in tasks performed by physicians and paramedical staff). Duties relegated to paramedical staff consisted primarily of "health care services," which involved counseling and health education, and "preventive maintenance services" (as opposed to the "sick care services" provided by various primary-care physicians and other medical specialties) (Garfield et al. 1976). Such adjustments enabled this HMO to provide greater access to services for substantially more patients. The model, essentially an industrial engineering solution to the uncertain needs of each patient entering the system, appears to have met with a positive response from both staff and

Figure 9.1 Medical Care Delivery System

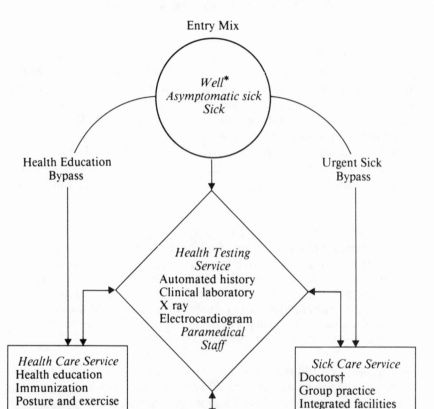

Source: Garfield et al. 1976. Reprinted by permission of *The New England Journal of Medicine* 294(1976): 427.

*Includes worried well.
†Solo or group practice.

patients. Well-conceived bureaucratic models can be more responsive to the needs of patient and staff than less self-consciously thought-out professional structures.

Professional Structure. New health practitioners have frequently been used to enhance the productivity of traditional physician practices and to support professional modes of organization. Physician assistants are typically best equipped, because of their training in medical schools, to serve such objectives. Often, they work with an individual physician or small primary group practice, and, in terms of their activity patterns in such practices, function like physicians. Physician assistants tend to have brief encounters with patients, performing more tests than physicians and providing little in the way of patient education (Smith and Morris 1980).

> I enjoy the work, but it's not easy fitting into the pattern of an existing practice. A lot of times it doesn't work out, and physician assistants move around a lot. The hours are long and sometimes I feel a little exploited. We get the duller and more difficult side of medicine and the pay pales in comparison (George Johnson, army medical corpsman and graduate of the Duke University Physician's Assistant for a General Practitioner program in rural North Carolina).

An appropriately utilized physician assistant can increase the productivity of a physician by as much as 70 percent. That translates into a significant increase in physicians' incomes in practices where demand will absorb this extra capacity. The vision of a physician supervising half-a-dozen assistants in a busy practice frightens most third parties, who fear the exponential increase in the volume of charges that such practices could generate; in fact, most third parties restrict payments for such assistants. In spite of the lure of shorter working hours and higher net income, physicians have been slow to hire "physician extenders." In part this is because of the malpractice questions that such a practice raises, and in part it is because of the increasing supply of physicians, which has made the ability of any individual physician to expand his or her volume of visits more problematic. Mostly, however, it results from the difficulty physicians have with integrating such practitioners into a professional mode of organization. It is difficult to balance the degree of autonomy needed for such practitioners to assure their optimum use with the supervisory responsibilities of the physician; many physicians do not feel comfortable with such a style of practice.

Participatory Structure. New health practitioners have also been used in a variety of settings to establish a more egalitarian, collaborative relationship between the patient and the practitioner. Nurse practitioners in primary-care settings, for example, emphasize patient education and preventive care. They spend extended periods with patients establishing such a relationship and in some cases are utilized in home-care settings. Nurse midwives perhaps illustrate the extreme in terms of developing a participatory relationship with clients. Nurse midwifery is a development of the childbirth education movement, which has radically changed patterns of childbirth in this country (Wertz and Wertz 1977).

> "I worked six years in obstetrics after I got my R.N. I felt frustrated. I only saw the mothers for a couple of days while they were hospitalized. When they left, I'd lose touch. Now I can follow them for almost a year. It's more satisfying for both of us. . . . When I started working on an obstetric unit in 1963 it was so different. All the mothers were knocked out. We used large doses of Demerol and Phenergan and, on top of that, Scopolamine. Scopolamine creates amnesia, so the mothers can't remember what happened afterwards. It also was a very disorienting effect. I can remember when we were very busy, I caught a woman crawling out of the delivery room on her hands and knees. She said she had to go to the bathroom. She delivered a few minutes later. It was crazy. I got experience with obstetrics though. We would do everything for the mothers and the doctors would arrive to catch the baby. Sometimes they didn't get there in time.
>
> Today, we work differently. The parents make a lot of the decisions, even siblings are permitted to participate in the birth in some circumstances. The choice of anesthesia and location of delivery is left up to them. We supply them with the information and help participate in the decision. Instead of whisking the baby away, the baby can remain with the mother. We now have a clearer idea how important that is. We stay with the mother throughout the whole process, helping her to understand what's happening, coaching, and supporting her. We spend a lot of time with our mothers, it's a tight, close relationship. I think it's important to them, I know I find it far more fulfilling than the kind of assembly line relationship I had with them as a nurse in the earlier days before I became a midwife nurse practitioner and before all the changes in hospital deliveries took place" (nurse midwife, in Zimmerman and Smith 1980, 64–75).

Alternatives on the Intermediate Level

Health maintenance organizations are the fastest growing segment of the health sector and the most visible intermediate level solution being offered. As we have described previously, many persons have argued that, through the discipline of a fixed, capitation payment system, HMOs represent the most appropriate mechanism for rationalizing and rationing health services. There are, however, a variety of ways that such organizations can be structured.

Professional Structure. One form of HMO, developed initially as a defensive measure by local medical societies, is the independent practice association (IPA). It allows member physicians to continue to treat patients in their private offices and pays them either on a capitation or fee basis. The IPA, in turn, enrolls subscribers in a comprehensive benefits plan, including physician and hospital services. The IPA assures physicians, through its board and structure, of control. Just as with other forms of group practice, however, the IPA has not always proved successful; practitioners are reluctant to give up the autonomy they must in order to assure adequate cost controls. Plans that fail to assure such controls meet quick but painful deaths.

The Rise and Fall of Healthwatch

The impending development of a Kaiser-type HMO in Rochester galvanized the local medical community into action. "We can offer the same services, and people can keep their own physicians," was the response, motivated both by pride and by a fear of losing income. Unfortunately, the physicians learned too late what would be required to make such a seemingly effortless plan work. Their lack of attention to selective enrollment risks and internal utilization controls doomed Healthwatch. It offered the same benefits as the HMO, and at a comparable price. Enrollment began on the same date. Healthwatch jumped to a quick lead in the battle for enrollment. Local physicians leaped to the support of the medical society's plan, placing advertising posters for Healthwatch in their own waiting rooms (a practice not unlike advertising for auto insurance in a body shop). Then the impact of their utilization experience began to hit. Their number of hospital days was 50 percent above that of conventional Blue Cross coverage. When this difference was added to the premiums of the plan, enrollment plunged by more than half in six months. Those left were persons most likely to add more than their share to the costs. It soon became clear that the plan was no longer viable. Healthwatch folded, amid heated accusations and finger pointing.

Bureaucratic Structure. The latest entries into the HMO market have been locally developed HMOs acquired by CIGNA and other insurance-based conglomerates in the Fortune 500. There has been little attempt as yet to centralize the management of these diverse holdings, but the model of choice is the Kaiser system. In such a plan, physicians share some of the risks associated with the operation, since some of their income derives from bonuses paid out of whatever surplus remains at the end of a particular fiscal period. The structure clearly involves a resource-constraining approach. For example, the Kaiser plans operate with about 1.5 hospital beds per 1,000 enrollees, in contrast to the 4.5 per 1,000 national average, and with about 80 physicians per 100,000 enrollees, as opposed to about 160 physicians per 100,000 persons in the general population. Physician extenders are used, in a structure somewhat like that described for the micro level, to assure that costly hospital and physician resources are used efficiently.

Participatory Structure. Many of the early versions of HMOs established by labor unions and neighborhood health centers had elements of a participatory structure. Medical and other staff are involved in nontraditional outreach programs that involve health education and even food programs. There is a more open-ended commitment to patients. Care is more likely to be organized by teams, combining as much as possible health aides, nurses, and physicians on an equal basis in discussions of case management; families also have a greater role.

ONLOK

ONLOK, a capitation-based HMO for a nursing home-eligible population, is based in a high-rise apartment complex for the elderly (which it also owns) in the Chinatown section of San Francisco. A community-controlled, nonprofit corporation, ONLOK has attracted widespread attention and has been widely imitated. Its board is composed of community people, and the chairman is a respected leader in Chinatown. The organization has arranged for a waiver for their capitation plan enrollees from Medi-Cal and Medicare. Instead of fee-for-service payments, they are paid a lump sum, blended capitation payment from these two sources, which comes to somewhat less than the cost per day in an area nursing home. The organization hires its own staff, including a physician, pharmacist, physical therapist, occupational therapists, and nurse practitioners. Enrollees participate in a day-care program at a community center, which, in addition to typical recreational activities, provides all the health and personal care services one might receive in a nursing home. Enrollees are then returned to their families for the evening. ONLOK's widespread acceptance in the community and its apparent cost-effectiveness has not, however, left it without critics. Many local physicians are hostile to the plan, in part because of the capitation mechanism and in part because of the physicians' loss of authority in the management of patients, which in ONLOK is shared with the nurses and caseworkers (Gottesman 1984).

Alternatives on the Macro Level

The idea of rationing health services is receiving growing acceptance. External controls give providers a budget, or at least a fixed, predictable stream of utilization or income that they can count upon in developing a budget. There are many ways of organizing so that such rationing can be achieved.

Professional Structures.

Whether the Feds are interested primarily in cost or in quality, you can expect them to continue to push controls whenever they're paying the bills. "It's going to be more like kids in high school grading each other's papers," observes North Carolina pediatrician Glenn A. Kiser. "But perhaps that's better than having an armchair sociologist doing it" (Dekker 1976, 106).

The "If we don't do it, somebody else will and we won't like it" ethic has motivated most initial efforts to control costs. Only when professional self-policing has clearly failed has it been possible to impose external controls on the medical profession. Such self-policing or rationing through utilization review has proved effective in controlling expenditures in some situations. For example, internal peer review has proved effective in reducing the number of normal tonsils and appendixes removed in a hospital (Donabedian, Axelrod, and Wyszewianski 1980, 268, 276).

Some IPAs, such as the San Joaquin Medical Foundation, have mounted effective utilization review mechanisms that have reduced utilization and kept premiums at a competitive level. The PROs and their predecessors, the Professional Standards Review Organizations, which were developed from early, successful peer review experiences and made a requirement of the Medicare program, have not been as clearly effective at controlling costs (Health Care Financing Administration 1980). Such controls work best with the full cooperation of practitioners, and that cooperation comes only with a clearly and universally perceived threat to income and professional autonomy.

Bureaucratic Structures. Multi-institutional systems, many persons have argued, can efficiently ration resources and thereby provide greater overall cost savings and efficiency. Whether public, as in the case of the Veterans Administration, or private, as in the case of investor-owned chains, these systems have similar opportunities for rationing resources and for monitoring their use. In an investor-owned chain, the administrator of the local facility is typically faced with a set of financial goals.

Hospital Corporation of America

Hospital Corporation of America (HCA), based in Nashville, Tennessee, is now the largest of the hospital management companies. It began in the late 1950s, in part because of the efforts of cardiologist Thomas Frist, who with the help of some colleagues built his own facility, Park View Hospital, by selling shares to raise the capital. HCA now has 391 hospitals with 56,144 beds. This includes ownership of acute-care hospitals in the United States (almost 170), management of acute-care facilities and psychiatric facilities in the United States, and ownership of acute-care facilities outside the country. Gross revenues were $3.9 billion in 1983, up 11 percent over 1982, and each bed earned well over $2,000 (Standard and Poors 1983, Hospital Corporation of America 1983). This profit appears to have been earned by maintaining (1) higher occupancy through physician marketing and recruitment efforts, (2) somewhat lower nurse-to-patient ratios, and (3) higher prices (relative to their voluntary counterparts) for ancillary services for their predominantly charge-paying clientele.

According to some observers, HCA's approach to competition appears to have been, "Don't waste dollars to compete, use the dollars to acquire" (Wohl 1984, 117). The company has rapidly absorbed potentially competitive chains and has acquired indirect control of others through stock ownership. It has also attempted to purchase a teaching hospital affili-

ated with Harvard University and has provided special subsidies for research programs at about a half-dozen university-
based health administration programs. This same effort to
diversify and vertically integrate services has resulted in its
acquisition of home health agencies and a recent effort to
merge with American Hospital Supply.

Proponents argue that the development of such systems and the
budgetary control they are able to exercise over their operations translate into greater efficiency and cost control for the health system as a
whole. The translation is done by competitive market forces, which protect the consumer, at least in the long run, from price gouging and substandard care. All that needs to be done is to alter the way firms are
paid to assure that they have an incentive to provide care efficiently.

The most recent attempt to create a competitive market has been
the implementation of the DRG pricing system for the Medicare program. Many observers, aware of the inflated charges in investor-owned
chains, expected that DRGs might take the wind out of the proprietar-
ies' sails. If there is any lesson to be learned from the proprietary nursing home sector, it is that this is unlikely to happen. The production-
oriented approach to payment fits the bureaucratic model of organizing
services well and provides an attractive incentive to investor-owned
chains: it requires relatively minor adjustments in operations.

It is doubtful, however, that DRGs will be able to control costs of
the system as a whole. Demand for hospitalization is highly variable
among communities. There is a more than threefold variation in hyster-
ectomy rates in Maine, for example, and many other DRG categories
exhibit even greater regional differences. It should be relatively easy to
influence such rates of admission, however, either through marketing
aimed at existing medical staff or recruitment of additional physicians.
While cost per unit of service may be controlled, more units of service
will be provided and thus overall system costs will continue to increase
(Wennberg, McPherson, and Caper 1984).

Participatory Structures. As in industry, participatory approaches
in the field of health care appear to be the last resort. Physicians and
administrators will embrace such approaches only when professional or
bureaucratic controls become onerous or obviously fruitless and when
the ability of physicians and facilities to survive under those controls is
clearly threatened. The basic approach is simple: create a decentralized
budgeting process and let each local facility work out its own way of living within these constraints while meeting the needs of its particular
constituency. It seems reasonable to assume that whoever has to live

within these constraints is best able to devise ways of minimizing their adverse impact. The discipline that is imposed by a well-developed budgeting process within an institution is imposed on all health services within a geographic area.

Such a budgetary system appears to have worked well within the Veterans Administration (VA). While it is difficult to make direct comparisons, the capital equipment budgets of VA facilities appear to be less than one-tenth those of comparable community hospitals in the same region (Halpern 1984). A similar approach, although limited to payments to acute-care hospitals, has been taken in Rochester, New York, and among some facilities in the Finger Lakes region of New York. A maxicap, "the total sum of dollars the community is willing to spend during a given period on hospital care," is established in negotiations between such third parties as Medicaid, Medicare, and Blue Cross and representatives of the hospitals and the community (Sigmond 1986). Two other decisions that need to be made someday by a representative community group are (1) what goods and services should be purchased with this fixed set of funds and (2) how these funds should be dispersed to the particular hospitals.

While the formulas that have been devised for paying operating and capital expenditures in the Rochester plan provide only relatively modest cost savings and appear to provide no adequate incentives for cooperative planning among facilities, they do appear to provide a framework for more effective cost control than the professional and bureaucratic models we have described. The plan is similar to that of the Swedish model described in chapter 1 and, lest the idea seem alien, identical to the operation of local school boards throughout the United States. Some of these ideas have been incorporated in recent national health insurance proposals.

We could provide many other illustrations of the influence these organizational assumptions have on the structuring of innovations. The general drift, however, at all three levels, has been toward more bureaucratic (larger, greater centralization, and greater specialization), privately owned structures. Does this make sense? Before we attempt to answer the question, let us review what we know about the effect of structure on performance.

THE IMPACT OF STRUCTURE
ON PERFORMANCE

Structure has two distinct impacts on the performance of an organization. First, structure affects the internal efficiency of an organization.

Second, it affects the relative degree of influence and control the organization can exert over its external environment. We reviewed the research on the relationship between structure and internal efficiency in chapter 3, and we described the relationship between organizational structure and the power an organization exerts over its external environment in chapter 6. We need only summarize those conclusions here.

Internal Advantages

Evidence from research has raised questions about what contribution the basic structural changes in the health sector have made to the efficient production of services.

1. Increased size of organizations: In general, economies of scale appear to be extremely modest or nonexistent. Clear diseconomies of scale exist in particularly large medical practices (more than five physicians) and in large facilities (more than 400 beds).

2. Increased centralization: Combining units into multi-institutional systems has consistently produced higher operational costs.

3. Specialization: Increased specialization appears to consistently add to overall costs.

4. Privatization: Proprietary acute-care hospitals appear to cost third parties more, while proprietary nursing homes appear in general to cost less than their nonprofit counterparts. These differences reflect differences in the reimbursement incentives in the two sectors and, consequently, the greater responsiveness of proprietary facilities to financial incentives. Whether this would translate into greater system efficiency, given the appropriate incentives, is questionable.

In other words, the evidence suggests that the increases in organizational size, centralization of control, specialization, and private ownership have, on balance, significantly reduced the efficiency with which services are provided.

External Advantages

As we have suggested, the first choice of any organization facing a problem (particularly if it has to do with internal efficiency) is not to attempt to improve performance, but to manipulate the external environment. If the organization can exercise sufficient power over its environment, it need make no adjustments at all. While recent structural changes have done very little to improve organizational performance, they have made organizations exceptionally well able to exercise power over their environments. As we suggested in chapter 6, other things being equal:

1. The larger the organization, the greater its power over its environment. The organization can exert that power to negotiate more advantageous conditions with the professionals it employs, the third parties from which it receives payment, or the market it serves.

2. The higher the degree of specialization, the greater control an organization is able to exert over its environment. The organization's ability to attract patients becomes less dependent on what has been described as the "lay referral network" and more dependent on its relationship to professionals or other organizations. The more specialized the organization, the more likely it is to be able to control information and knowledge, insulating itself from external influence in the classic manner that professions do. Specialization and the division of labor associated with it also enable the organization to exert greater bureaucratic control over staff. Such specialization enables the organization to substitute more unskilled and semiskilled employees for autonomous, more professional employees.

3. The more centralized the organization is, the greater its power over its environment. A multi-institutional system is in a far better position to negotiate with a state Medicaid program, for example, than are independent operators held together only loosely by a trade association.

4. Private ownership offers more power over the environment than does voluntary or public ownership. Privately owned organizations have a variety of options (such as changing services, relocating, and so on) that are not available to voluntary or publicly owned organizations.

These relationships are well understood and are usually listed as major advantages of developing multi-institutional systems (Ermann and Gabel 1984). Administrators are attracted to these shifts since they make the kind of services offered, to whom, and where more managerial decisions, unencumbered by local community interests or concerns. This flexibility is recognized in financial circles, making it far easier and less expensive for such organizations to gain access to capital markets. As access to capital becomes more restricted and as reimbursement policies make the financial viability of individual institutions more problematic, these advantages are increased.

The external advantages we have presented clearly outweigh the advantages of internal efficiency and have stimulated most of the shifts in structure that have taken place. It is ironic that these shifts, which have resulted in the erosion of community and public control, have been stimulated by public initiatives to finance and control health services (that is, by Medicaid and Medicare and the resulting efforts to control costs in these programs). It is also ironic that antitrust laws, which attempt to assure the vigorous, competitive free market that these newly emerging organizational structures value, have been a major obstacle to their development.

CONCLUSIONS

Choices in the organization and management of health services are not value-free. In fact, we have illustrated how various innovations in the delivery of health services can be structured to serve quite different interests and organizational models.

There have been massive changes not just in the structure of health care and in its scientific-technological base, but also in what it represents. Our society has moved from a diffuse, holistic conception of health care that emphasized the relationship between the patient and the community to a conception of health care as the responsibility of an elite, scientifically trained profession. It has since moved, as a result of the expanding scientific base and third-party payments, toward a conception of health care as simply another economic good, one that should be organized and treated just like any other. The shifting structure of the system reflects those changes. Are these shifts inevitable? Is it a sheer waste of effort to resist them? We have suggested a rational basis for resisting these changes: there appear to be inherent contradictions in them, contradictions that will eventually force some new kind of synthesis and, possibly, a restructuring of the system.

That new synthesis is being forced by dramatic changes in the way we think about how organizations work and how individuals can stay healthy or be cured of illnesses. Effective organizations and effective healing and prevention require a less mechanical, more participatory approach. The opportunity for such participation will be enhanced to the extent that the following tenets guide the structuring of health care organizations:

1. Decentralization: Decisions concerning the financing, licensure, standards, and planning of health services should be made at the lowest possible level. Decentralization helps reduce the power of professional and provider associations and erodes the advantage of multi-institutional systems that lack local community ownership; at the same time, it makes the public interest less diffuse. It also helps focus accountability, which is now spread out among individual providers; local, state, and federal bureaucracies; and third-party payers.

2. Miniaturization: Services should be provided in the smallest feasible units. Large institutions and group practices create centers of power that are more likely to be controlled by corporate or professional interests and less by consumers.

3. Desegregation: Consumers should be provided services in the least specialized and least restrictive settings consistent with good medical practice. The more a particular service or organization is shared by all members of a community, the stronger the influence it can exert.

4. Reappropriation: Services should be owned by those who use and, consequently, pay for them. That ownership, whether of a public facility or a voluntary community facility, does not rule out contracting for private management services as long as such services are directed toward community goals.

We are a long way from anything that follows such guidelines, but we suggest them here as an anchor against the drift resulting from too little critical evaluation. We have offered some support for these guidelines in the previous chapters, and we leave it to the reader to develop whatever compromise or contingency approach makes sense to him or her.

The structure of the system will eventually change in the direction we have outlined above, because fundamentally it is what we need—and because, when given a fair test, it will work. There is a hardy strain of rationality in the health care system, and this, along with the "gradual encroachment of ideas" against the power of vested interests, will bring about a change of direction. The change will result from small acts of courage and commitment on the part of individuals and organizations. It will be shaped by persons who are uncomfortable with the gap between what health care is and what it should be.

References

Alexander, J., and L. Morlock. 1985. "Multi-Institutional Arrangements: Relationships Between Governing Boards and Hospital Chief Executive Officers," *Health Services Research* 19: 675–99.

All the President's Men, film based on Woodward, Bob, and Carl Bernstein. 1974. *All The President's Men*. New York: Simon and Schuster.

American College of Surgeons. 1920a. "Hospital Standardization." *Surgery, Gynecology, and Obstetrics* 30: 641–47.

———. 1920b. "The Process of Hospital Standardization." *Surgery, Gynecology, and Obstetrics* 30: 543–44.

American Hospital Association. 1984. *Hospital Statistics*. Chicago: AHA, 4–6.

———. 1985. *Legal Issues in the Negotiation and Implementation of a Statute*. Chicago: AHA.

Anderson, J.B., and S.J. Jay. 1985. "Computers and Clinical Judgment: The Role of Physician Networks." *Social Science and Medicine* 20: 969–79.

Anderson, O., and R. Anderson. 1967. *A Decade of Health Services*. Chicago: University of Chicago Press.

Andrews, J. 1973. "Medical Care in Sweden: Lessons for America." *Journal of the American Medical Association*. 223: 1373.

Apt, Joan. 1983. Blue Cross of Greater Philadelphia. Personal communication, November.

———. 1984. Blue Cross of Greater Philadelphia. Personal communication, September.

Asch, S.E. 1952. *Social Psychology*. Englewood Cliffs, N.J.: Prentice-Hall.

Asher, C. 1984. "Impact of Social Networks on Adult Health." *Medical Care* 22: 349–459.

Barash, Daniel S. 1984. "Lou Gehrig, David Niven and Me." *The Village Voice* 29(16): 1, 12–15.

Becker, M. 1970. "Sociometric Location and Innovativeness: Reformation and Extension of the Diffuse Model." *American Sociological Review* 35: 267–83.

Berliner, Howard S. 1975. A Larger Perspective on the Flexner Report. *International Journal of Health Services* 5: 573–90.

———. 1984. Scientific Medicine Since Flexner." In *Alternative Medicines*, ed. J. Warren Salmon. New York: Tavistock, 30–56.

Berne, E. 1963. *The Structure and Dynamics of Organizations and Groups.* Philadelphia: J.B. Lippincott.

———. 1964. *Games People Play.* New York: Grove Press.

Bicknell, R. 1977. Personal communication.

Birnbaum, H., C. Bishop, A.J. Lee, and G. Jenson. 1981. "Why Do Nursing Home Costs Vary? The Determinants of Nursing Home Costs." *Medical Care* 19: 1095–1107.

Blackstone, Irwin. 1977. "The AMA and the Osteopathic Study on the Power of Organized Medicine." *Antitrust Bulletin* 22 (Summer): 405–40.

Blake, R., and J. Mouton. 1967. "Organizational Excellence Through Effective Management Behavior." *Manage* 20(2): 42–47.

Blumberg, M. 1980. "Health Status and Health Care Use by Type of Private Health Care Coverage." *Health and Society: Milbank Memorial Fund Quarterly* 58: 633–55.

Broida, L., M. Lerner, F. Lohrenz, and F. Wenzel. 1975. "The Impact of HMO Membership in an Enrolled Prepaid Population on Utilization of Health Services in a Group Practice." *New England Journal of Medicine* 295: 780–83.

Brook, R.H., J.E. Ware, and W.H. Rogers. 1983. "Does Free Care Improve Adults' Health?" *New England Journal of Medicine* 309: 1426–34.

Brown, M., and B.P. McCool. 1980. *Multihospital Systems.* Germantown, Md.: Aspen Systems Corp.

Bucher, R., and J.G. Stelling. 1977. *Becoming Professional*, vol. 46. Beverly Hills, Calif.: Sage Publications.

Bunker, J.P., J. Fowles, and R. Schaffarzick. 1982. "Evaluation of Medical-Technology Strategies: Effects of Coverage and Reimbursement." *New England Journal of Medicine* 306: 620–24.

Burling, T., E. Lentz, and R. Wilson. 1956. *The Give and Take in Hospitals.* New York: G.P. Putnam's Sons.

Burns, Lawton R. 1982. "The Diffusion of Unit Management among U.S. Hospitals." *Hospital and Health Services Administration* 27(2): 43–57.

Burns, Linda A. 1981. "Hospital Initiatives in Response to Reductions in Medicaid Funding for Ambulatory Care Programs." Working paper, American Hospital Association, Chicago.

Caplan, G. 1974. *Support Systems and Community Mental Health: Lectures on Concept Development.* New York: Behavioral Publications.

Carroll, Lewis. 1946. *Alice in Wonderland and Through the Looking Glass.* New York: Grosset & Dunlap.

Carroll, Marjorie Smith, and Ross H. Arnett III. 1981. "Private Health Insurance Plans in 1978 and 1979: A Review of Coverage, Enrollment and Financial Experience." *Health Care Financing Review* 3(1): 55–88.

Cochrane, A. 1972. *Effectiveness and Efficiency.* London: The Nuffield Provincial Hospitals Trust.

Cohen, M.D., J.G. March, and J.P. Olsen. 1972. "A Garbage Can Model of Organizational Choice." *Administrative Science Quarterly* 17: 1-25.

Coser, R.L. 1962. *Life in the Ward.* East Lansing, Mich.: Michigan State University Press.

Cousins, Norman. 1979. *Anatomy of an Illness As Perceived by the Patient.* New York: W.W. Norton.

Crichton, M. 1970. *Five Patients: The Hospital Explained.* New York: Alfred A. Knopf.

Cristoffel, T. 1976. "Medical Care Evaluation." *Journal of Medical Education* 51: 83-88.

Cromwell, Jerry, and James Kanak. 1982. "The Effects of Prospective Reimbursement Programs on Hospital Adoption and Service Sharing." *Health Care Financing Review* 4(2): 67-88.

Crutchfield, Richard S. 1955. "Conformity and Characters." *American Psychologist* 10: 191-98.

Dabbs, James M., and Irving L. Janis. 1965. "Why Does Eating While Reading Facilitate Opinion Change?" *Journal of Experimental and Social Psychology* 1: 133-44.

Davis, Karen, and Diane Roland. 1983. "Uninsured and Underserved: Inequities in Health Care in the United States." *Health and Society: Milbank Memorial Fund Quarterly* 61: 149-76.

Davis, Karen, Marsha Gold, and Diane Makuc. 1981. "Access to Health Care for the Poor: Does the Gap Remain?" *Annual Review of Public Health* 2: 159-82.

Davis, Loyal. 1960. *Fellowship of Surgeons: A History of the American College of Surgeons.* Springfield, Ill.: Charles C. Thomas.

Dekker, Marianne G. 1976. "If Peer Review Won't Work, What Will?" *Medical Economics.* 17 May, pp. 101-2, 106.

Doctor X. 1965. *Intern.* New York: Harper & Row.

Doherty, N., J. Segal, and B. Hicks. 1978. "Alternatives to Institutionalization for the Aged: Viability and Cost Effectiveness." *Aged Care and Services Review* 1(1): 1-16.

Donabedian, Avedis, Solomon Axelrod, and Leon Wyszewianski. 1980. *Medical Care Chartbook,* 7th ed. Washington, D.C.: AUPHA Press.

Dorazio, Leo. 1984. Personal communication.

Dowling, Alan F. 1980. "Do Hospital Staff Interfere with Computer System Implementation?" *Health Care Management Review* 5(4): 23-58.

Downs, A. 1967. *Inside Bureaucracy.* Boston: Little, Brown.

Downs, G.W., and L.B. Mohr. 1979. "Conceptual Issues in the Study of Innovation." *Administrative Science Quarterly* 21: 700-714.

Dubois, P. 1967. "Organizational Visibility of Group Practice." *Group Practice* 16: 261-70.

Ebert, Robert. 1973. "The Medical School." *Scientific American* 229(3): 138-50.

Eggers, P. 1980. "Risk Differential Between Medicare Beneficiaries Enrolled and Not Enrolled in an HMO." *Health Care Financing Review* 4 (Winter): 91-99.

Ellwood, Paul. 1974. *Alternatives to Regulation: Improving the Market.* Minneapolis: Interstudy.

Enthoven, A.C. 1978. "Shattuck Lecture: Cutting Cost Without Cutting Quality of Care." *New England Journal of Medicine* 298: 1229–38.

Ermann, D., and J. Gabel. 1984. "Multi-hospital Systems: Issues and Empirical Findings." *Health Affairs* 3(1): 50–64.

Etzioni, Amitai. 1961. *A Comparative Analysis of Complex Organizations.* New York: Free Press of Glencoe.

Evans, Robert. 1982. "A Retrospective on the 'New Perspective.'" *Journal of Health Politics, Policy and Law* 7(2): 325–44.

Eyer, J. 1977. "Does Unemployment Cause the Death Rate to Peak in Each Business Cycle? A Multifactor Model of Death Rate Change." *International Journal of Health Services* 7: 1625–62.

Falk, I.S., M.C. Klem, and N. Sinai. 1933. *The Incidence of Illness and the Receipt and Costs of Medical Care among Representative Family Groups.* Committee on the Costs of Medical Care report no. 26. Chicago: CCMC.

Feder, Judith, Jack Hadley, and Ross Mullner. 1984. "Falling Through the Cracks: Poverty, Insurance Coverage, and Hospital Care for the Poor, 1980 and 1982." *Health and Society: Milbank Memorial Fund Quarterly* 62: 544–66.

Feder, J.M., and W. Scanlon. 1980. "Regulating the Bed Supply in Nursing Homes." *Health and Society: Milbank Memorial Fund Quarterly* 58: 54–87.

Feldstein, P.J. 1977. *Health Associations and the Demand for Legislation: The Political Economy of Health.* Cambridge, Mass.: Ballinger.

Fennell, M.L. 1984. "Synergy, Influence and Information in the Adoption of Administrative Innovations." *Academy of Management Journal* 27(1): 113–29.

Fisher, George Ross. 1980. *The Hospital That Ate Chicago.* Philadelphia: Saunders.

Flood, A., W. Scott, and W. Ewy. 1984. "Does Practice Make Perfect? Part II: The Relation Between Volume and Outcomes and Other Hospital Characteristics." *Medical Care* 22: 113–23.

Freedman, Jonathan L., and Scott C. Fraser. 1966. "Compliance Without Pressure: The Foot-in-the-Door Technique." *Journal of Personality and Social Psychology* 4: 195–202.

Freidson, Eliot. 1970. *Profession of Medicine: A Study of the Sociology of Applied Knowledge.* New York: Dodd, Mead.

Freshnock, L.J., and L.J. Goodman. 1979. "Medical Group Practice in the United States: Patterns of Survival Between 1969 and 1975." *Journal of Health and Social Behavior* 20: 352–62.

Friedman, Milton. 1962. *Capitalism and Freedom.* Chicago: University of Chicago Press.

Fuchs, Victor R. 1974. *Who Shall Live?* New York: Basic Books.

Galbraith, Jay R. 1982. "Designing the Innovating Organization." *Organizational Dynamics* 10 (Winter): 5–25.

Gamson, W.A. 1968. *Power and Discontent.* New York: Holt, Rinehart & Winston.

Ganey, T. 1978. "Sikeston's Firm Nursing Homes Get More Funds." *St. Louis Post Dispatch.* 14 May, p. 1.

Garfield, Sidney R., Morris F. Collen, Robert Feldman, Krikor Soghikian, Robert Richart, James B. Duncan. 1976. "Evaluation of an Ambulatory Medical-Care Delivery System." *New England Journal of Medicine* 294: 426–31.

Gartner, Alan, and Frank Riessman. 1974. *The Service Society and the Consumer Vanguard.* New York: Harper & Row.

Gaus, C., B. Cooper, and F. Hirschman. 1976. "Contrasts in HMO and Fee-for-Service Performance." *Social Security Bulletin* 39(5): 3–14.

Gaus, Clifton, and Norman Fuller. 1972. "HMO Evaluation: Utilization Before and After Enrollment." Paper presented at the American Public Health Association annual meeting, Atlantic City, 13–16 November.

General Accounting Office. 1983. "Hospital Merger Increased Medicare and Medicaid Payments for Capital Costs." GAO publication no. HRD-84-10. Washington, D.C.: Government Printing Office.

Getzen, Thomas E. 1981. "Quality, Reputation and Transaction of Patients: An Economic Analysis of Medical Group Practice." Ph.D. diss., University of Washington, Seattle.

———. 1984. "The Relationship Between Income and Health Expenditures." Working paper, Department of Health Administration, Temple University, Philadelphia.

Gibson, Robert M., Daniel R. Waldo, and Katharine R. Levit. 1983. "National Health Expenditures, 1982." *Health Care Financing Review* 5(1): 1–31.

Ginzberg, Paul B., and Daniel M. Koretz. 1983. "Bed Availability and Hospital Utilization: Estimates of the 'Roemer Effect.' " *Health Care Financing Review* 5(1): 87–92.

Glaser, B.G., and A.L. Strauss. 1970. "Dying on Time." In *Where Medicine Fails,* ed. A. Strauss. New York: Aldine, pp. 131–42.

Goldsmith, S. 1984. *Theory Z Hospital Management: Lessons from Japan.* Rockville, Md.: Aspen Publications.

Goodman, L.J., E.H. Bennett, and R.J. Odem. 1976. *Group Medical Practice in the U.S.* Chicago: American Medical Association.

Gordon, James S. 1984. "Holistic Health Centers in the United States." In *Alternative Medicines,* pp. 229–87. *See* Berliner 1984.

Gottesman, Len. 1984. Personal communication.

Gray-Toft, P., and J. Anderson. 1985. "Organizational Stress in the Hospital: Development of a Model for Diagnosis and Prediction." *Health Services Research* 20: 753–74.

Greenberg, Jill. 1982. "The Fight for Safety and Health at the Workplace." *Consumer Health Perspectives* 8 (6): 1–8.

Greer, A.L. 1984. "Medical Technology and Professional Dominance Theory." *Social Science and Medicine* 18: 809–17.

Griffith, John R. 1972. Letter to the editor. Association of University Programs in Health Administration, *Program Notes* 43 (December): 12–13.

Hadley, Jack. 1982. *More Medical Care, Better Health?* Washington, D.C.: Urban Institute Press.

Hage, J. 1974. *Communications and Organizational Control.* New York: John Wiley and Sons.

Hage, J. 1980. *Theories of Organizations: Form, Process, and Transformation.* New York: Wiley-Interscience.

Hage, J., and M. Aiken. 1967. "Program Change and Organizational Properties: A Comparative Analysis." *American Journal of Sociology* 72: 503–19.

Hage, J., and R. Dewar. 1973. "Elite Values Versus Organizational Structures in Predicting Innovation." *Administrative Science Quarterly* 18: 279–90.

Halberstam, M. 1971. "The Doctor's New Dilemma—Will I Be Sued?" *New York Times Magazine.* 14 February, pp. 8–9, 33–37.

Hall, Oswald. 1948. "Stages of a Medical Career." *American Journal of Sociology* 53: 327–36.

Halpern, Jay. 1984. District coordinator, District Four, Veterans Administration Medical Center, Philadelphia. Personal communication.

Hasenfeld, Yeheskel. 1983. *Human Service Organizations.* Englewood Cliffs, N.J.: Prentice-Hall.

Havighurst, C. 1976. *Competition in a Regulated Health Care System.* Washington, D.C.: Federal Trade Commission.

Health Care Financing Administration. 1980. "Professional Standards Review Organization 1979 Program Evaluation." In *Health Care Financing Research Report*, HCFA publication no. 03041. Washington, D.C.: Government Printing Office.

Health Care Financing Review. 1985. 6(3): 14.

Health Services Research Center. 1977. "Services Shared by Health Care Organizations." Chicago: Hospital Research and Educational Trust and Northwestern University.

Hefty, T. 1969. "Returns to Scale in Hospitals: A Critical Review of Research." *Health Services Research* 4: 267–80.

Hemminkis, Z., and A. Paakkulainen. 1976. 'The Effects of Antibiotics on Mortality from Infectious Diseases in Sweden and Finland." *American Journal of Public Health* 66: 1180–84.

Hirschman, A.O. 1970. *Exit, Voice, and Loyalty.* Cambridge, Mass.: Harvard University Press.

Hooyman, N., and J. Kaplan. 1976. "New Roles for Professional Women: Skills for Change." *Public Administration Review* 4: 374–78.

Hospital Corporation of America. 1983. *Annual Report.* Nashville, Tn.: HCA.

"Hospital Indicators." 1981. *Hospitals* 55(13): 39–42.

"Hospital Statistics." 1971. *Hospitals*, guide issue. 45(15): 460–62.

Ingram, Deborah, Diane Makuc, and Joel C. Kleinman. 1986. "National and State Trends in Use of Prenatal Care 1970–73." *American Journal of Public Health* 76: 415–23.

Institute of Medicine. 1985. *Preventing Low Birthweight.* Washington, D.C.: National Academy Press.

Intercollegiate Case Clearing House. N.d. *Sunrise Hospital: A Case in Innovative Marketing Strategy.* Publication 9-578-691. Boston: ICCH, mimeographed.

Jackson-Beeck, Marilyn, and John H. Kleinman. 1983. "Evidence of Self-Selection among Health Maintenance Organization Enrollees." *Journal of the American Medical Association* 250: 2826–29.

James, J. 1974. "Impacts of the Medical Malpractice Slow Down in Los Angeles County: January 1976." *American Journal of Public Health* 69: 437–43.

Janis, Irving L., Donald Kaye, and Paul Kirschner. 1965. "Facilitating Effects of 'Eating-While-Reading' on Responsiveness to Persuasive Communications." *Journal of Personality and Social Psychology* 1: 181–85.

Johnson, Miriam M., and Harry W. Martin. 1958. "A Sociological Analysis of the Nurse Role." *American Journal of Nursing* 58: 373–77.

Joskow, P.L. 1981. *Controlling Hospital Costs.* Cambridge, Mass.: MIT Press.

Kaluzny, Arnold D. 1982. "Quality Assurance As a Managerial Innovation: A Research Perspective." *Health Services Research* 17: 253–68.

Kaluzny, A.D., and J.E. Veney. 1977. "Types of Change and Hospital Planning Strategies." *American Journal of Health Planning* 1(3): 13–19.

Kaluzny, A.D., J.E. Veney, and J.T. Gentry. 1974. "Innovation of Health Services: A Comparative Study of Hospitals and Health Departments." *Health and Society: Milbank Memorial Fund Quarterly* 52: 51–82.

Kaluzny, A.D., J.E. Veney, J.T. Gentry, and J.B. Sprague. 1971. "Scalability of Health Services: An Empirical Test." *Health Services Research* 6: 214–23.

Kanter, Rosabeth Moss. 1983. *The Change Masters.* New York: Simon and Schuster.

Kaplan, H.B. 1967. "Implementation of Program Change in Community Agencies." *Milbank Memorial Fund Quarterly* 45 (July): 321–31.

Katz, Daniel, and Robert L. Kahn. 1978. *The Social Psychology of Organizations,* 2nd ed. New York: John Wiley & Sons.

Kelman, S. 1973. Personal communication.

Keynes, John Maynard. 1936. *The General Theory of Employment, Interest, and Money.* London: MacMillan and Co.

Kidder, David, Gary Gaumer, and Stephen Mennemeyer. 1981. *Review and Synthesis of Research Findings on the Distribution and Effectiveness of Health Care Manpower.* Washington, D.C.: U.S. Department of Health and Human Services, Public Health Service.

Kiewsler, C. 1982. "Mental Hospitals and Alternative Care: Noninstitutionalization as Potential Public Policy for Mental Patients." *American Psychologist* 37: 349–60.

Kimberly, J.R. 1978. "Hospital Adoption of Innovation: The Role of Integration into External Informational Environments." *Journal of Health and Social Behavior* 19: 361–73.

Kinzer, David M. 1959. "The Only Team that Pilots and Doctors Recognize Is Their Own." *Modern Hospital* 92(5):59–65.

Kisch, A., and A. Viseltear. 1967. *The Ross-Loos Medical Group.* Medical Care Administration case study no. 3. Arlington, Va.: U.S. Department of Health and Human Services, Public Health Service.

Kjerulff, Kristen H. 1982. "Predicting Employee Adaptation to the Implementation of a Medical Information System." In *Proceedings: Sixth Annual Symposium on Computer Applications in Medical Care*, ed. Bruce I. Blum. New York: Institute of Electrical and Electronics Engineers, pp. 392–97.

Kjerulff, Kristen H., Michael A. Counte, Jeffrey C. Salloway, Bruce C. Campbell. 1983. "Measuring Adaptation to Medical Technology." *Hospital and Health Services Administration* 28 (January–February): 30–40.

Kovner, Anthony, 1974. Personal communication.

Kuttner, Robert. 1985. "Blue-Collar Boardrooms: A Practical Look at Everyone's Favorite Industrial Panacea." *The New Republic.* 17 June, 18–23.

Landefeld, J., and E. Seskin. 1982. "The Economic Values of Linking Theory to Practice." *American Journal of Public Health* 72 (6): 555–66.

Lee, A.J., and H. Birnbaum. 1983. "The Determinants of Nursing Home Operating Costs in New York State." *Health Services Research* 18 (Part 2): 285–308.

Lee, K., N. Paneth, L.M. Gartner, M.A. Pearlman, and L. Gruss. 1980. "Neonatal Mortality: An Analysis of the Recent Improvement in the United States." *American Journal of Public Health* 70: 15–21.

Lewin, Laurence S., Robert A. Derzon, and Rhea Margulies. 1981. "Investor-Owneds and Nonprofits Differ in Economic Performance." *Hospitals* 55(13): 52–58.

Luft, Harold S. 1981. *Health Maintenance Organizations: Dimensions of Performance.* New York: John Wiley & Sons.

McClure, W. 1981. "Structure and Incentive Problems in Economic Regulation of Medical Care." *Health and Society: Milbank Memorial Fund Quarterly* 59: 107–44.

McElrath, D. 1961. "Perspectives and Participation of Physicians in Prepaid Group Practice." *American Sociological Review* 26: 596–607.

McGuirk, Marjorie, and Frank W. Porelli. 1984. "Spatial Patterns of Hospital Utilization: The Impact of Distance and Time." *Inquiry* 21: 84–95.

McKelvey, Bill. 1982. *Organizational Systematics, Taxonomy, Evolution, Classification.* Berkeley: University of California Press.

McKinney, M. 1984. "The Newest Miracle Drug: Quality Circles in Hospitals." *Hospital and Health Services Administration* 29(5): 74–87.

McNaughton, D.C. 1981. (Chairman of the Board, Health Corporation of America.) Advertisement in the *Wall Street Journal.* 23 January, p. 8.

McNeil, K., and E. Miniham. 1977. "Medical Technology Regulations and Organizational Change in Hospitals." *Administrative Science Quarterly* 22: 475–90.

McPhee, John. 1984. "Heirs of General Practice." *New Yorker.* 23 July, pp. 40–85.

Manning, W.G., A. Leibowitz, G.A. Goldberg, W.H. Rogers, and J.P. Newhouse. 1984. "A Controlled Trial of the Effect of a Prepaid Group Practice on Use of Services." *New England Journal of Medicine* 31: 1505–10.

March, J., and H. Simon. 1964. *Organizations.* New York: John Wiley & Sons.

Martin, Suzanne, Michael Schwartz, Bernadette J. Whalen, Debra D'Arpa, Greta M. Ljung, John Holden Thorne, Anne E. McKusick. 1982. "Impact of a Mandatory Second-Opinion Program on Medicaid Surgery Rates." *Medical Care* 20: 21–39.

Maslow, Abraham H. 1943. "A Theory of Human Motivation." *Psychological Review* 50: 370–96.

Mechanic, David. 1962. "Sources of Power of Lower Participants in Complex Organizations." *Administrative Science Quarterly* 7: 349–64.

Meiners, M. 1982. "Nursing Home Costs: A Statistical Cost Function Analysis Using National Survey Data." Ph.D. diss., Georgetown University, Washington, D.C.

Mintzberg, Henry. 1979. *The Structuring of Organizations: A Synthesis of the Research.* Englewood Cliffs, N.J.: Prentice-Hall.

———. 1983. *Power In and Around Organizations.* Englewood Cliffs, N.J.: Prentice-Hall.

Mitchell, Janet B. 1978. "Patient Outcomes in Alternative Long-Term Care Settings." *Medical Care* 16: 439–52.

Mitchell, J.H., and J. Dunn. 1978. "Comparative Absence Experience among Employees Covered by a Prepaid or BC/BS Health Insurance Program." *Journal of Occupational Medicine* 20: 797–800.

Moch, M., and E. Morse. 1977. "Size, Centralization and Organizational Adoptions of Innovations." *American Sociological Review* 42: 716–25.

Mohr, Lawrence B. 1969. "Determinants of Innovation in Organizations." *American Political Science Review* 43 (March 1969): 111–26.

Mohr, Lawrence B. 1971. "Organizational Technology and Organizational Structure." *Administrative Science Quarterly* 16 (December): 444–59.

Morse, Edward V., Gerald Gordon, and Michael Moch. 1974. "Hospital Costs and Quality of Care: An Organizational Perspective." *Health and Society: Milbank Memorial Fund Quarterly* 52: 315–46.

Myers, Beverlee. 1983. "Equity: A Governmental Perspective." In *The Question of Equity,* ed. Sondra S. Cooney. Durham, N.C.: Duke University Department of Health Administration and Duke Endowment, pp. 112–23.

Mytinger, R.E. 1968. *Innovation in Local Health Services.* Public Health Service publication no. 1164-2. Washington, D.C.: Government Printing Office.

Nadler, D.A. 1977. *Feedback and Organizational Development: Using Data-Based Methods.* Reading, Mass.: Addison-Wesley.

Nathanson, C.A., and Laura Morlock. 1980. "Control Structure, Values and Innovation." *Journal of Health and Social Behavior* 21: 315–33.

National Center for Health Statistics. 1979. (Augustine Gentile.) *Physician Visits: Volume and Interval Since Last Visit, U.S.—1975.* Series 10, data from the National Health Survey no. 128, DHEW publication no. (PHS) 78-1556. Washington, D.C.: Government Printing Office.

———. 1981. (Alvin Sirrocco.) *Employees in Nursing Homes in the United States: 1977 National Nursing Home Survey.* Series 14, data from the National Health Survey no. 25, DHHS publication no. 81-1820. Washington, D.C.: Government Printing Office.

———. 1983. (J.G. Collins.) *Physician Visits: Volume and Interval Since Last Visit, United States, 1980*. Series 10, no. 144, DHHS publication no. (PHS) 83-1572. Washington, D.C.: Government Printing Office.

———. 1984. (E.J. Graves.) *1983 Summary: National Hospital Discharge Survey*. Advance data from Vital and Health Statistics no. 100, DHHS publication no. (PHS) 84-1250. Washington, D.C.: Government Printing Office.

National Physicians Committee. 1946. *Compulsion: The Key to Collectivism*. Chicago: NPC.

Newhouse, Joseph P., Willard G. Manning, Carl N. Morris, Larry L. Orr, Naihua Duan, Emmett B. Keeler, Arleen Leibowitz, Kent H. Marquis, M. Susan Marquis, Charles E. Phelps, Robert H. Brook. 1981. "Some Interim Results from a Controlled Trial of Cost-Sharing Health Insurance." *New England Journal of Medicine* 305: 1501-7.

New York Times. 1984. 11 July, p. 1.

Ng, Sik Hung. 1980. *The Social Psychology of Power*. New York: Academic Press.

Nourian, Ed. 1978. Personal communication.

Ouchi, W.G. 1977. "Relationship Between Organizational Structure and Organizational Control." *Administrative Science Quarterly* 22: 95–113.

———. 1981. *Theory Z: How American Business Can Meet the Japanese Challenge*. Reading, Mass.: Addison-Wesley.

Owens, A. 1979. "Doctor's Earnings: A Brighter Picture This Time." *Medical Economics*. 15 September, pp. 118–31.

Palmer, R.H., and M.C. Reilly. 1979. "Individual and Institutional Variables Which May Serve as Indicators of Quality of Medical Care." *Medical Care* 17: 693–717.

Palola, Ernest G., and Joseph F. Jones. 1965. "Contrasts in Organizational Features and Role Strains Between Psychiatric and Pediatric Wards." *Journal of Health and Human Behavior* 6: 155–63.

Palumbo, D. 1969. "Power and Role Specificity in Organizational Theory." *Public Administration Review* 29: 237–48.

Pattison, Robert V., and Hallie M. Katz. 1983. "Investor-Owned and Not-for-Profit Hospitals." *New England Journal of Medicine* 309: 347–53.

Pear, R. 1985. "Decline Slowing in Infant Death Rates." *New York Times*. 24 February, p. 1.

Pelz, D.C., and F.C. Munson, 1980. "A Framework for Organizational Innovating." Paper presented at the Academy of Management annual meeting, Detroit, 9–13 August.

———. 1982. "Originality Level and the Innovating Process in Organizations." *Human Systems Management* 3: 173–87.

Perrow, C. 1963. "Goals and Power Structures: A Historical Case Study." In *The Hospital in Modern Society*, ed. E. Freidson. New York: Free Press of Glencoe, pp. 112–46.

Peter, L.J., and R. Hull. 1967. *The Peter Principle*. New York: Bantam Books.

Peters, Thomas J., and Robert H. Waterman, Jr. 1982. *In Search of Excellence: Lessons from America's Best-Run Companies*. New York: Basic Books.

Pfeffer, J. 1981. *Power in Organizations.* Marshfield, Mass.: Pitman Publishing.

Prugh, D.G., E. Staub, H. Sands, R. Kirschbaum, and E. Lenihan. 1953. "A Study of the Emotional Reactions of Children and Families to Hospitalization and Illness." *American Journal of Orthopsychiatry* 22: 70–106.

Quint, Jeanne. 1972. "Institutionalized Practices of Information Control." In *Medical Men and Their Work*, ed. Eliot Freidson and Judith Lorber. New York: Aldine-Atherton, pp. 220–38.

Reinhardt, Uwe. 1984. "The Health Professions' Collision Course." *Hospitals* 58 (16): 96–97.

Relman, Arnold. 1984. "Who Will Pay for Medical Education in Our Teaching Hospitals?" *Science* 226: 20–23.

Rhee, Sang-O. 1983. "Organizational Determinants of Medical Care Quality: A Review of the Literature." In *Organization and Change in Health Care Quality Assurance*, ed. D.L. Roice, J.C. Krueger, and R.E. Modrow. Rockville, Md.: Aspen Publications.

Rice, Dorothy. 1978. "Projection and Analysis of Health Status Trends." Paper presented at the American Public Health Association annual meeting, Los Angeles, 15–19 October.

Rice, Dorothy P., Thomas A. Hodgson, and Andrea N. Kopstein. 1986. "The Economic Cost of Illness: A Replication and Update." *Health Care Financing Review.* Forthcoming.

Ries, W. 1974. "Journal for Social Psychology of Hospitals." Sloan Institute of Hospital Administration, Cornell University.

Roemer, Milton I., and William Shonick, 1973. "HMO Performance: The Recent Evidence." *Health and Society: Milbank Memorial Fund Quarterly* 51: 271–317.

Romeo, Anthony A., Judith L. Wagner, and Robert H. Lee. 1984. "Prospective Reimbursement and Diffusion of New Technologies in Hospitals." *Journal of Health Economics* 3: 1–24.

Roos, L.L., and F.A. Starke, 1981. "Organizational Roles." In *Handbook of Organizational Design*, vol. 1, ed. P. Nystrom and W. Starbuck. Oxford: Oxford University Press, pp. 290–308.

Rosen, George. 1977. "Contract or Lodge Practice and Its Influence on Medical Attitudes to Health Insurance." *American Journal of Public Health* 67: 374–78.

Rosner, David. 1982. *A Once Charitable Enterprise: Hospitals and Health Care in Brooklyn and New York 1985–1915.* New York: Cambridge University Press.

Rosner, Martin M. 1968. "Administrative Controls and Innovation." *Behavioral Science* 13: 36–43.

Ruchlin, Hirsch S., Madelon L. Finkel, and Eugene G. McCarthy. 1982. "The Efficacy of Second-Opinion Consultation Programs: A Cost-Benefit Perspective." *Medical Care* 20: 3–20.

Rundall, Tom, and Wendy K. Lambert. 1984. "The Private Management of Public Hospitals." *Health Services Research* 19: 518–44.

Russell, L.B. 1979. *Technology in Hospitals.* Washington, D.C.: The Brookings Institution.

Sager, A. 1983. "Why Urban Voluntary Hospitals Close." *Health Services Research* 18: 451–75.

Salkever, D.S., and T.W. Bice. 1976. "The Impact of Certificate of Need Controls on Hospital Investment." *Health and Society: Milbank Memorial Fund Quarterly* 54: 185–214.

Salmon, J. Warren. 1984. "Defining Health and Reorganizing Medicine." In *Alternative Medicines*, pp. 252–88. *See* Berliner 1984.

Saward, Ernest. 1976. Personal communication.

Saxe, John Godfrey. 1979. "The Blind Men and the Elephant." *The Illustrated Treasury of Poetry for Children.* New York: Grosset and Dunlap, p. 232.

Schein, E.H. 1972. *Organizational Psychology*, 2nd ed. Englewood Cliffs, N.J.: Prentice-Hall.

Scheirer, M.A. 1981. *Program Implementation: The Organizational Context.* Beverly Hills, Calif.: Sage Publications.

Scott, W.R., A.B. Flood, and W. Ewy. 1979. "Organizational Determinants of Services, Quality and Cost of Care in Hospitals." *Health and Society: Milbank Memorial Fund Quarterly* 57: 234–64.

Shain, Max, and Milton Roemer. 1959. "Hospital Costs Relate to Supply of Beds." *Modern Hospitals* 92 (April): 71–74.

Shattuck, L., N.P. Banks, Jr., and J. Abbott. 1850. *Report of the Sanitary Commission of Massachusetts.* Boston: Dutton and Wentworth State Printers. Reprinted in 1948 by Harvard University Press.

Sheff, T.J. 1961. "Control over Policy by Attendants in a Mental Hospital." *Journal of Health and Social Behavior* 1: 93–105.

Shem, Samuel. 1978. *The House of God.* New York: Dell.

Shortell, Stephen M. 1982. "Theory Z: Implications and Relevance for Health Care Management." *Health Care Management Review* 7(4): 7–21.

Shortell, Stephen M., Selwyn W. Becker, and Duncan Neuhauser. 1976. "The Effects of Management Practices on Hospital Efficiency and Quality of Care." In *Organizational Research in Hospitals*, ed. Stephen M. Shortell and Montague Brown. Chicago: Blue Cross Association, 90–107.

Sigmond, Robert M. 1986. Personal communication.

Sirrocco, Alvin. 1981. *Employees in Nursing Homes in the United States: 1977 National Nursing Home Survey.* National Center for Health Statistics series 14, no. 25, DHHS publication no. 81-1820.

Slater, Philip. 1970. *The Pursuit of Loneliness: American Culture at the Breaking Point.* Boston: Beacon Press.

Smith, David Barton. 1970. "St. Joseph Hospital Survey." Ithaca, N.Y.: Sloan Institute of Hospital Administration, Cornell University.

———. 1981. *Long-Term Care in Transition: The Regulation of Nursing Homes.* Washington, D.C.: AUPHA Press.

Smith, David Barton, and Arnold D. Kaluzny. 1974. "Inequality in Health Care Programs: A Note on Some Structural Factors Affecting Health Care Behavior." *Medical Care* 12: 860–70.

Smith, David Barton, and Steve Morris. 1980. "Physician Extender Practice Activity Patterns." Working paper, Health Care Financing Administration, Office for Research Development Services.

Sorensen, Andrew A., Richard P. Wersinger, Klaus J. Roshmann, J. William Gavett. 1979. "A Note on the Comparison of the Hospital Cost Experience of Three Competing HMOs." *Inquiry* 16: 167–71.

Spitzer, Walter A., David L. Sackett, John C. Sibley, Robin S. Roberts, Michael Gent, Dorothy J. Kergin, Brenda C. Hackett, Anthony Olynich. 1974. "The Burlington Randomized Trial of the Nurse Practitioner." *New England Journal of Medicine* 290: 251–56.

Standard and Poors. 1983. "Health Care, Hospitals, Drugs and Cosmetics: Prospective Payments To Alter Industry." *Standard and Poors Industry Surveys.* New York: Standard and Poors, sect. 2.

Stebbins, M.W., J.A. Hawley, and A.L. Rose. 1982. "Long-Term Action Research: The Most Effective Way to Improve Complex Health Care Organizations." In *Organizational Development in Health Care Organizations*, ed. N. Margulies and J.D. Adams. Reading, Mass.: Addison-Wesley, pp. 105–36.

Steinberg, Sam. 1984. Personal communication.

Stevens, Rosemary A. 1983. "Equity: The Issue." In *The Question of Equity*, pp. 25–33. *See* Myers 1983.

Stone, Katherine. 1974. "The Origins of Job Structure in the Steel Industry." *Review of Radical Political Economics* 6(2): 113–73.

Stumpf, G.B. 1976. "Why Some HMOs Develop Slowly." *Public Health Reports* 91 (November-December): 496–503.

Sudnow, D. "Dead on Arrival." In *Where Medicine Fails*, pp. 111–29. *See* Glaser and Strauss 1970.

Temkin-Greener, H. 1983. "Interprofessional Perspectives on Team Work in Health Care: A Case Study." *Health and Society: Milbank Memorial Fund Quarterly* 61: 641–58.

Terris, M. 1976. "The Epidemiologic Revolution, National Health Insurance and the Role of Health Departments." *American Journal of Public Health* 66: 1155–64.

Thomas, L. 1983. *The Youngest Science: Notes of a Medicine-Watcher.* New York: Bantam Books.

Thomsen, R. 1975. *Bill W.* New York: Harper & Row.

Toffler, A. 1969. *Future Shock.* New York: Bantam Books.

Treat, T.F. 1976. "Performance of Merging Hospitals." *Medical Care* 14: 199–209.

U.S. Department of Commerce, Bureau of the Census. 1979. *Statistical Abstract of the U.S., 1978.* Washington, D.C.: Government Printing Office.

U.S. Department of Health and Human Services. 1984. *Health United States and Prevention Profile 1983.* Washington, D.C.: Government Printing Office.

U.S. Department of Health and Human Services. 1985a. Press release. 31 July.

U.S. Department of Health and Human Services. 1985b. *Projections of Physician Supply in the United States.* Office of Data Analysis and Management report no. 3-85, HRP-0906330. Washington, D.C.: Government Printing Office.

U.S. Department of Health, Education, and Welfare. 1978. *Current Medicare Survey Report.* DHEW publication no. MBR-1 (11-78). Washington, D.C.: Government Printing Office.

Varela, J. 1971. *Psychological Solutions to Social Problems.* New York: Academic Press.

Vignola, Margo L. 1979. "Economics of Excess Hospital Capacity." Paper presented to the Medical Care Section of the American Public Health Association annual meeting, 8 November.

Wagner, David. 1980. "The Proletarianization of Nursing in the United States 1932–1965." *International Journal of Health Services* 10: 271–90.

Wall Street Journal. 1981. 12 August, p. 46.

Wall Street Journal. 1985. 8 March, p. 33.

Walton, R.C. 1969. "Two Strategies of Social Change and Their Dilemmas." In *Planning of Change,* ed. W. Bennis, K.D. Benne, and R. Chin. New York: Holt, Rinehart & Winston, pp. 167–75.

Warner, D. 1973. "Allocation Within Large, Decentralized Public Firms: The Case of the New York Hospital System." Working paper no. 15, Health Services Research Program, Yale University Institution for Social and Policy Studies, New Haven, Conn.

Warner, K.A. 1975. "A 'Desperation-Reaction' Model of Medical Diffusion." *Health Services Research* 10: 369–83.

Watt, J.M., R.A. Derzon, S.C. Renn, C.J. Schramm, J.S. Hahn, and G.D. Pillari. 1986. "The Comparative Economic Performance of Investor-Owned Chain and Not-for-Profit Hospitals." *New England Journal of Medicine* 314: 89–96.

Weber, Max. 1947. *Theory of Social and Economic Organization,* trans. Talcott Parsons. New York: Free Press.

Weick, K.E. 1969. *The Social Psychology of Organizing.* Reading, Mass.: Addison-Wesley.

Weiner, Myron, and Troy Caldwell. 1981. "Stresses and Coping in ICU Nursing." *General Hospital Psychiatry* 3: 119–227.

Weisfeld, N., and D. Falk. 1983. "Choosing Elusive Competence." *Hospitals* 57(5): 61–68.

Weiss, James E., and Merwyn R. Greenlick. 1970. "Determinants of Medical Care Utilization: The Effects of Social Class and Distance on Contacts with the Medical Care System." *Medical Care* 8: 456–62.

Wennberg, John E., and Alan M. Gittelsohn. 1982. "Variations in Medical Care among Small Areas." *Scientific American* 246(4): 120–35.

Wennberg, John E., Kim McPherson, and Philip Caper. 1984. "Will Payment Based on Diagnosis-Related Groups Control Hospital Costs?" *New England Journal of Medicine* 311: 295–300.

Wertz, Richard W., and Dorothy C. Wertz. 1977. *Lying In: A History of Childbirth in America.* New York: Free Press.

Whyte, William Foote. 1948. *Human Relations in the Restaurant Industry.* New York: McGraw-Hill.

Whyte, William Foote, Tove Helland Hammer, Christopher B. Meek, Reed Nelson, Robert N. Stern, eds. 1983. *Worker Participation and Ownership.* New York: ILR Press, State School of Industrial and Labor Relations, Cornell University, Ithaca.

Wieland, G., and A. Bradford. 1981. "An Evaluation of the Hospital Internal Communication (HIC) Project. In *Improving Health Care Management*, ed. G. Wieland. Ann Arbor, Mich.: Health Administration Press.

Winslow, C.E. 1923. *The Evolution and Significance of the Modern Public Health Campaign.* New Haven, Conn.: Yale University Press.

Wohl, Stanley. 1984. *The Medical Industrial Complex.* New York: Harmony.

Wolfe, Tom. 1971. *Radical Chic and Mau-Mauing the Flak Catchers.* New York: Bantam Books.

———. 1979. *The Right Stuff.* New York: Farrar, Straus & Giroux.

Woollcott, Marie. 1961. "Verses."

Zaltman, G., and R. Duncan. 1977. *Strategies for Planned Change.* New York: Wiley-Interscience.

Zimmerman, Barbara, and David Barton Smith. 1980. *Careers in Health.* Boston: Beacon Press.

Zuckerman, Howard D. 1979. "Multi-institutional Systems: Promise and Performance." *Inquiry* 16: 291–314.

Index

126; power of, 179 (fig.); response
of pressure to change, 183–202, 184
(fig.); set, 124; structure of, effect
on change, 195–201; theater as an
analogy to, 124–34; transactions
within, 136
Other-directed systems, 186

Parent-bureaucrat orientation, 136
Participatory management, 107–8
Participatory structure, 235,
237–38, 240
Pastimes, 135
Patient's ability to heal self, 104–5.
See also Holistic health; Holistic
health centers
Peer Review Organizations, 51, 152,
238
Persuasion: curiosity in, 219; design
of, 214 (fig.); distraction in, 218; by
successive approximation, 214–15
Peter Principle, 126
Physician assistant, 234
Physician/population ratios in
HMOs, 62
Power, 156–61; distribution within
organizations, 160 (fig.);
expandable, 160 (fig.); expertise, as
element of, 161; fixed, 160, (fig.);
flow of in health care system, 156
(fig.); group, 165; of health services
organizations, 179 (fig.);
individual, 161–68; as limited or
unlimited resource, 159; position,
as an element of, 162; residual,
163; sources, 161; tactics of,
209–10; tactics combined with
attitude change, 221–24
Preferred provider organizations
(PPOs), 186, 190
Prepayment plans, sponsored by
hospitals, 172
Primary care nursing, 106
Privatization, 41–42, 178

Problem, recognition of, 191–93;
"Product-line management," 106
Professional Standards Review
Organization (PSRO), 239
Professional status, 16
Professional structure, 234, 236–39
Providers: primary, 17; secondary, 17;
shifts in patterns of control of,
177 (fig.)
Psychological approach toward
attitude change, 212
Public control, erosion of, 242–44
Public policy, strategy for controlling
health care system, 173

"Quality circles," 106, 226

Rate-setting groups, state, 174
Rationalized machine model of ideal
organization, 36
Reactance as a factor in attitude
change, 213
Regulatory approach to controlling
health care system, 173
Reimbursement: abuses, 59; in the
basis of DRGs, 60, 65, 68; fixed,
74; prospective, 195
Remunerative control mechanisms,
169–71
Research and development: effect on
health system, 57–58; in HMOs,
62–63
Residual power, 163
Rituals, 134–35
Role, 124
— conflict, 125
— overload, 128
— senders, 125
— set, 124; for nurse, 125 (fig.); for
director, 125 (fig.)
— theory, 134
Ross-Loos Medical Group, 22–23
Rousseau, 137

About the Authors

DAVID BARTON SMITH, M.A., Ph.D., is professor and chairman of the Department of Health Services Administration at Temple University. He has previously held faculty positions with the Graduate School of Management Sloan Program in Hospital Administration at Cornell University and in the Community Medicine Department at the University of Rochester School of Medicine. Dr. Smith has also served as an Intergovernmental Personnel Act Fellow for the Office of Policy and Research in the Health Care Financing Administration, a consultant to the Institute of Medicine on Nursing Home Regulation and to The Robert Wood Johnson Foundation program on Health Care Cost Containment. He has served as chairman of the Philadelphia Health System Agency's advisory task force on organ transplants and currently serves on the board of Booth Maternity Hospital in Philadelphia. Dr. Smith is the author of several books and numerous articles. He received his master's degree in social science from Michigan State University and his doctorate in medical care organization from The University of Michigan.

ARNOLD D. KALUZNY, M.H.A., Ph.D., is a professor in the Department of Health Policy and Administration, School of Public Health, University of North Carolina at Chapel Hill. He is also a clinical professor in the School of Pharmacy and a senior research associate at the University of North Carolina Health Services Research Center and the Lineberger Cancer Center. He is a consultant to a number of private research corporations and various international, federal, and state agencies, including the World Health Organization, the National Cancer Institute, the National Heart, Lung, and Blood Institute, the National Center for Health Services Research and Technology Assessment, and the Office of Medical Research Applications of the National Institutes of Health. He is the author of numerous articles and co-author of several books, including *Health Care Management: A Text in Organizational Theory and Behavior* with Stephen M. Shortell and *Evaluation Design Making for Health Services Programs* with James E. Veney. Dr. Kaluzny received his master's degree in hospital administration from The University of Michigan Graduate School of Business Administration and his doctorate in medical care organization from The University of Michigan.